TRAUMA JUNKIE

TRAUMA JUNKIE

Memoirs of an Emergency Flight Nurse

JANICE HUDSON

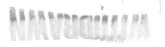

FIREFLY BOOKS

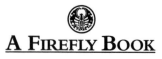

A FIREFLY BOOK

Published by Firefly Books Ltd. 2001

First Printing

U.S. Cataloging-in-Publication Data
(Library of Congress Standards)

Hudson, Janice
  Trauma junkie : memoirs of an emergency flight nurse / Janice Hudson. – 1st ed.
[240] p. : col. ill. ; cm.
Includes index.
Summary : Personal experiences of a former CALSTAR (San Francisco area)
emergency flight nurse.

ISBN 1-55209-503-7 (bound)
ISBN 1-55209-573-8 (pbk.)

1. Emergency medical services – Personal narrative. 2. Rescue work – United States –
Personal narrative. 3. California Shock Trauma Air Rescue (CALSTAR). I. Title.
362.18/ 092 21 2001 CIP

Canadian Cataloguing in Publication Data

Hudson, Janice, 1959-
  Trauma Junkie : memoirs of a flight nurse

ISBN 1-55209-503-7 (bound)
ISBN 1-55209-573-8 (pbk.)

1. Hudson, Janice, 1959-   . 2. Emergency medical personnel – California –
San Francisco – Biography. 3. Nurses – California – San Francisco – Biography.
I. Title.

RT37.H77A3 2001   610.73'092   C00-932615-4

Published in Canada by
Firefly Books Ltd.
3680 Victoria Park Avenue
Willowdale, Ontario M2H 3K1

Published in the United States by
Firefly Books (U.S.) Inc.
P.O. Box 1338, Ellicott Station
Buffalo, New York 14205

Design by Interrobang Graphic Design Inc.
Printed and bound in Canada by Friesens, Altona, Manitoba

*The Publisher acknowledges the financial support of the Government of Canada through
the Book Publishing Industry Development Program for its publishing activities.*

Introduction

IN 1987, I left a full-time job in the Seton Medical Center emergency department to take a position with California Shock/ Trauma Air Rescue (CALSTAR), an air ambulance service in the San Francisco Bay Area. At the time, this was an emerging field, and CALSTAR was only three years old. I became enamored with the flying, and though I continued to do shift work in the ER, that was only a sideshow. My true love was the helicopter.

After three years in the air, I attended a stress debriefing class that was developed to help medical professionals cope with the awful spectacles we face on the job. One of the suggestions was to keep a journal as a way of dealing with the emotional pain. So I started to write, then I wrote some more. Stories started pouring out on paper. At first they were the horrible flights, usually involving children. Then came the amazing calls, the ones with remarkable circumstances or unusual interventions. Finally there were the ludicrous stories, the ones that were so absurd we came home laughing. I enjoyed my little hobby, and slowly the material began to pile up.

In 1996, I felt it was time to grow up and get a real job. Somehow I couldn't see being fifty and still making a living scraping drunks off the freeway. With the support of my husband, Mark, I returned to graduate school and after two nightmarish years, emerged with a Master's degree in nursing, specializing in anesthesia. I am now a full-time certified registered nurse anesthetist (CRNA). I love my new profession; but I still wistfully remember those wonderful years with CALSTAR.

I miss the breakneck pace of caring for critical trauma patients, and I miss the people I worked with. The relationships we shared were absolutely professional, yet intensely intimate at the same time. CALSTAR became an extended family, complete with bratty brothers and occasional spats that put us all on edge. Our work brought us all very close together in a sort of club that no one could really understand unless they had been part of it.

All the stories that follow are true, though some of the names and places have been changed for confidentiality. I hope they will give readers a glimpse of what the club was like.

Janice Hudson
January 2001

Lifting Off

I had the fear. The all-encompassing fear. That sickening, sinking feeling that the events unfurling before me were barreling rapidly out of my control. At any moment, the beeper would signal the end of this charade, this idea I might someday join the ranks of the best of the best, the elite of the nursing world. Flight nurses.

The helicopter was quiet for now. Morning preflight was done, and Harry had gone back into quarters to start the day's paperwork. The smell of Jet A fuel wafted through the hot July air. Our trauma bag was safely secured with the seat belt on the Day-Glo orange litter, and the tubing for the blood pressure monitor was coiled and stowed so it would be ready to use with one tug. The EKG patches, already attached to the cable, were set to be slapped onto our patient's chest. We were ready for anything. The only thing missing was some unfortunate soul who required our services. For a brief moment, I had a fantasy that maybe I could do this job after all.

Suddenly the pager vibrated on my belt. My stomach felt as if I were on the roller coaster from hell and my sweating hands shook as I grabbed the beeper, pushed buttons randomly and inadvertently deleted the message. My first act, and I had screwed it up.

My career as a flight nurse was off to an inauspicious start.

Harry, one of my mentors during training and my partner that first day, came loping out to the helicopter with Pete, our pilot, running close behind. "All right, let's go," he yelled as he swung into the front seat and effortlessly locked in with the four-point belt. "Ya all set?" he asked, reaching for the maps.

"Harry, I'm not ready. I erased everything on my pager. I don't even know where we're going."

"Now, just relax and take a deep breath," Harry said as I panicked. "I'm right here, and I'll help you. We're going to Santa Cruz County on Skyline Boulevard for a motorcycle accident." Pete cranked up the two jet engines, drowning out any further conversation until the intercom was powered up.

As we lifted off I froze, entirely forgetting everything I had learned in our radio class. Despite a week devoted to learning the system we used in the helicopter, and the various county frequencies, it was all now a complete blank. The nurses had four different radios to manage and the pilot three—seven frequencies that might be blaring all at the same time.

I squinted down at the radio console's millions of small buttons and switches. Harry reached over and switched my station to the dispatch radio to let them know of our liftoff time and ETA to the scene. He smiled and patted my hand.

There is a specialized language used on the radios, and I

certainly hadn't mastered it. I tentatively keyed up the mike to our dispatch. "Uh, CALSTAR One, this is CALSTAR, uh, base. I mean, this is CALSTAR One. We, uh, just took off—uh, *lifted* off from Concord."

There was a slight pause as dispatch considered my garbled message, and I could hear snickering in the background. "CALSTAR One, *we* are the base. *You* are the helicopter. And *you* are responding to a motorcycle accident on Skyline Boulevard. Your map coordinates are Thomas Brothers, page 64, B4. Your ground contact will be Captain 61 on fire white, frequency 154.280. Do you have an ETA?"

I was unsuccessfully trying to write down all of this essential information when I realized I had no idea what our ETA might be. Keying up the transmit button instead of the intercom button, I said, "Pete, they want to know what our ETA is."

Dispatch responded wryly. "CALSTAR One, you hit transmit instead of intercom."

"Oh, sorry."

Pete was up front, giggling. "Janice, relax. It's going to be sixteen minutes if the coordinates I have are correct."

Now I had to do my arithmetic. Let's see. It was 11:12. In sixteen minutes it would be, well, uh …

Harry again came to my rescue. "Base, CALSTAR One. We have an ETA of 11:28. Copy map coordinates and ground frequency. Confirm Valley Medical is open and willing to accept?"

"Open and accepting," base responded.

The first part of the flight hadn't gone well, but I was determined to get something right. As we approached the scene, I carefully dialed in our ground frequency and rehearsed the dialogue in my mind. I confidently switched off from the dispatch radio and onto the ground unit. "Captain 61, this is CALSTAR. We have an ETA of 11:28. Please let us know when you have a visual on us." Quite pleased with myself, I sat back and awaited their response.

"CALSTAR One, Captain 61. Your landing zone is going to be—"

Abruptly, his radio transmission was drowned out by traffic on two other concurrently running radios. One was a paramedic giving a lazy radio report to another hospital: "…and we have him on four liters of O_2, and are giving an Allupent nebulizer…" This traffic competed with the comm radio, which was also blaring: "Cherokee 654 Bravo, turn into left downwind after departure. Traffic in the pattern is a Cessna at your two o'clock."

I reached over to switch off the distracting radios, and succeeding in turning them all off. Including our ground contact. Desperation set in. "Harry, help me. I just turned off all the radios back here," I pleaded.

He reached over and flipped up the correct switch. "You're doing fine," he lied. "Takes a while to learn to work the mighty Wurlitzer. Now all you need to do is get our landing zone instructions. Piece of cake."

Despite my ineptitude, I did manage to get our LZ information from the fire department, who were already on scene. We were to land in a field about one mile away from the actual incident, as there were no safe LZs nearby. A fire truck was waiting to transport us to the accident. Pete circled the area and gently settled us onto the ground. "You're cleared out," he said. As I scrambled out of the helicopter, I remembered to buckle my seat belt behind me so I could find it quickly when we returned with the patient. Harry grabbed the trauma bag and together we scrambled up into the cab of the fire truck.

"Hey," Harry greeted the firefighters. "How's it going?"

"It's pretty crazy up here," one replied. "We now have two separate accidents less than a mile apart. You guys are getting the MCA patient, who planted his face into the back of a parked van while he was going about seventy miles an hour. No helmet—he's pretty messy. The ambulance that was supposed to respond to this accident had to stop up the road for the other one. I don't know if a second ambulance can get to this one."

I was only vaguely listening to this conversation. The fire truck ride was a hoot, and I was grinning like an idiot as we bounced along the rutted road, reflecting on what an enormously cool job this was. As we turned onto Skyline, the firefighter switched on the lights and siren to get through the backed-up traffic. I saw a sign that indicated we were leaving Santa Cruz County and entering San Mateo.

Harry groaned. "So this incident is actually in San Mateo, huh?"

"Yup," the firefighter said. I vaguely wondered what difference that made. "Well, here we are."

Out the window, a group of firefighters huddled around a supine figure on a backboard. We climbed out of the huge truck and trotted over to our patient. "Oh, Jesus," I said softly. This poor man wasn't recognizable as human. His head was a jagged mass of bone and tissue; his entire face was disconnected from his skull. Facial fractures are graded on the LaForte scale from one to four, depending how much of the face is still connected. This guy had a LaForte fifteen. One of the firefighters was vainly attempting to assist his breathing manually with a bag and mask, but I could tell it wasn't working well. Every time he gave the patient a breath, air would spurt out through holes in his forehead.

Harry asked me to take over the bagging, and the firefighter stood up and handed me the mask. Feeling a little squeamish, I knelt down to resume the impossible task. Because of his extensive facial trauma, there was no way to get an adequate seal on his face to force air into his lungs. I tried to readjust the mask several times, but it simply wasn't working. To make matters worse, with each breath I gave him, fine spray of blood squirted out and covered my trauma goggles, making it difficult to see.

"You guys got any portable suction? His airway is filled with blood, and we have to clear it out if we're going to get this guy tubed."

Intubating a patient is often among the first things EMS does on a scene, since a patient who can't breathe adequately on his own is at risk of brain damage within minutes. We put a lighted instrument called a laryngoscope into the mouth, pulling the tongue and epiglottis out of the way to locate the vocal cords at the entrance to the trachea. Then we insert a polyvinyl endotracheal tube (ETT) with a balloon at the end. Once this balloon is inflated, it creates a seal that prevents air from leaking out when we force a breath in with the bag. It also stops the patient from inhaling stomach contents if he vomits, a common scenario with a full belly. It's a crying shame for someone to survive the trauma, only to die of aspiration pneumonia two weeks later.

One of the firefighters returned with the suction, and Harry crouched by me as I was bagging. "When I open his mouth, hold his neck still," he said. "With this kind of impact, he's for sure got some injury to his neck. We don't want to complete a c-spine fracture and make him a quad."

I nodded and moved over to the side, gently holding our patient's head in neutral alignment. Harry knelt down and placed the laryngoscope in what was left of his mouth, trying to suction out the blood and debris and get a view of the vocal cords. "It's no use," he announced. "I can't see anything. Let's just get going."

Obediently, I took over bagging again and looked around. Under normal circumstances, there would be an ambulance there to take us back to the helicopter. But the paramedics were at the other accident and there was no place on the fire truck to put the patient. I had no idea what we could possibly do. The firefighters had finished strapping our patient to the backboard and were ready to go. But how? Harry, of course, had the whole thing figured out.

"I'll be back in a sec," he said, and jogged over to a man in a small black Toyota pickup stopped in traffic. "Excuse me, sir, but would you mind giving us a ride to our helicopter? It's about a mile down the road, and we really need to get there." The driver, speechless, just nodded his head. "OK, you guys. Load him up over here," Harry yelled, pointing to the back of the man's truck. Together we lifted the backboard and six of us piled into the bed of the truck. The fire engine cranked up and, with lights and siren, began escorting us through the massive backup. The driver of the pickup stared at us through the rearview mirror with eyes the size of saucers. He was rooted to the spot, and made no effort to move.

"Drive!" Harry shouted through the rear window, gesturing down the road. "Just drive! Follow the fire truck."

Our carjacked driver nodded vigorously, gunned the motor and shot out of the traffic, making all of us lose our balance and fall over. We lost our grasp on the backboard and our patient nearly slid off the open tailgate.

I'm gonna die, I thought. I'm gonna die before we get to the helicopter.

As we passed the sign to the county line, Harry pounded on the window of the cab. "Hey, could you pull over for a minute? I gotta do something." Our driver nodded and hit the brakes, causing us all to fall forward. Harry rummaged around in the trauma bag and pulled out the surgical kit, and before I could register, he had prepped the patient's neck and made an incision over the cricothyroid membrane. Air and blood rushed out, and Harry gently threaded in a trach tube. He grinned at me as he began to ventilate the patient with the first decent respirations since the accident.

"Neat trick, eh?" he said. "We're not authorized to do that in San Mateo, but we can in Santa Cruz. I had to wait till we got over the county line."

Harry turned to the driver again. "OK, we can go on now. You want to take a right on that dirt road up there." As we got to the aircraft and loaded him up, I reached down and felt for a radial pulse. It was reassuringly strong and regular. He was finally getting the oxygen he so desperately needed. We lifted off and had him in the trauma center in ten minutes.

I was just glad it was over.

This entire saga had started two months earlier, in May 1987, while I was in a restaurant in Tiburon overlooking San Francisco Bay. A friend of mine, Dana, was hosting a Sunday brunch celebrating my recent marriage. Mark was a co-worker in the ICU at Seton Medical Center, and our first date was purely out of mercy. I couldn't find anyone to go with me on a double date, and out of desperation I called him and begged. He only grudgingly agreed to go. At the time I thought he was gay—after all he was a cute male nurse from Texas with a great tush and a mustache. In San Francisco in the eighties, that usually meant gay. I found out that night he wasn't—to my surprise and delight.

Now I was sitting outside on the deck, enjoying the brilliant sunshine and sipping margaritas. "So what's this new job you have?" I asked as Dana mulled over the menu. Dana was another fellow nurse at Seton, and she was well known for seeking unusual jobs. She had worked in the emergency room, ICU, as a cruise ship nurse, and now she had started a position at California Shock/Trauma Air Rescue (CALSTAR), a non-profit helicopter air ambulance serving the Bay Area. It sounded intriguing.

"It's a new company in a relatively new industry," she explained, sipping her drink. "It's a dedicated EMS helicopter that responds to scenes, as well as doing a lot of interfacility flights—like getting people from a small hospital and taking them to the larger centers that can manage them. You know, stuff like cardiac, pediatrics, and trauma patients that find themselves at tiny rural hospitals. We're doing a lot of trans-ports for Children's Oakland."

But the most fun, she said, was the scene work. They'd fly out to accidents, scrape up the patients and try to get them to qualified care in that first "golden hour," when they'd have the best chance for meaningful survival after traumatic injuries. "A helicopter can really cut down on transport times. Besides, we can get them to specialized centers, too, that may be on the other side of the Bay—for things like burn care, spinal cord injuries, pediatric trauma. You'd love it."

"Do you carry a pager around and come in when some-thing happens?"

"Oh, no," she laughed. "We go to work and stay there for twenty-four-hour shifts. When we're activated, we're in the air within five minutes."

"So how many calls do you do per shift?"

"You might get none, or maybe five in a row. You never know. That's what makes it fun. Every day is something different, and most of the patients we transport are pretty sick, if not dead."

This really got me interested. Like Dana, I had already

worked in ICU and ER, and I seemed to gravitate to the most desperately ill. The work was intellectually challenging and often required rapid interventions, with little time to get bored. I realize now those were the early symptoms of adrenaline addiction, a condition identified many years later and common in paramedics, firefighters, police and other pre-hospital personnel.

I sent in my résumé and was invited for a formal interview. To my surprise, I was offered a job the following week and began the orientation in June—three mind-numbing weeks in a classroom and six weeks as a ride-along. Now I was finally ready to fly on my own. At least that's what they said. I wasn't so sure.

In those early weeks, while our new quarters were being built, CALSTAR was temporarily based out of the Sheraton Hotel in Concord, about twenty miles outside of Oakland. The crew was housed in two rooms, one for the pilot, and one for both nurses—the former filled with charts and maps, the latter with medical equipment.

I remember the awkward conversation Mark and I had about how my new job would impact our lives. "You'll be working twenty-four-hour shifts, huh?" he asked. "Guess that means you'll be sleeping at work."

"Sure will be strange not sleeping with you at night," I replied. "I'm going to miss you."

"So, uh, just where do you sleep at night? Guys in one room, girls in the other, like at camp?"

"I think the nurses sleep in one room and pilots in the other." There was a pregnant pause. "Are you OK with that?"

I was distinctly uneasy about the whole thing myself, now that I was actually faced with the prospect of sharing a room with Harry. Spending the night with a man I barely knew was bad enough; being in a hotel made it worse. And I was still mulling over a strange conversation I had had that morning with one of the other senior flight nurses, JoAnn, when she found out my first flight shift was to be with Harry.

"So do you know about him yet?" she had asked.

"Know about what?"

She leaned her head back and laughed. "You'll find out soon enough," she said, and walked away.

That afternoon, after we had finished cleaning up from our flight to Skyline Boulevard, I took a deep breath as I walked into our makeshift quarters.

"Well, well, well," Harry said. "That wasn't so bad, was it?"

Actually, I was exhausted from the ordeal and I settled into a chair, stretching out to admire my new boots and sleek black flight suit. The company had given me a hand-me-down from another flight nurse who had recently left, and it was a size too small. It would be another month or two until I got my own custom-tailored Nomex flight suits. I didn't care. I was delighted just to be here.

Not long after, the phone rang. It was dispatch, activating us to another motorcycle accident, or MCA, this one involving a train on the eastern reaches of Contra Costa County. Nervously, I ran out to the helicopter with Harry jogging along at my side.

"Ya ready?" he asked as we climbed into our seats and belted in.

My heart was pounding, and I could barely buckle my seat belt. "Yeah, um, sure. Now where are we going?"

"Deer Valley Road. Out behind Mount Diablo."

As far as I was concerned, it might have been Outer Mongolia. Like Steinberg's old *New Yorker* cartoon that shows the world more or less ending at the Hudson River, my knowledge of the Bay Area stopped at the San Mateo Bridge. All of the East Bay was a major mystery to me, and I only had a vague idea of the location of Mount Diablo—it was that peak you could see from San Francisco on a clear day.

As we circled the scene, I could see a group of firefighters huddled on the ground around a body on a backboard, next to a set of railroad tracks. The train was stopped, and the mangled remnants of a motorcycle were jammed under the front engine. Several railroad employees and a couple of firefighters were pulling on the motorcycle in a futile attempt to clear it from the track. We landed about a hundred yards away to avoid dusting off the group with our rotor wash.

Harry jumped out of the helicopter with the trauma bag and trotted over to the patient. I glanced over at the paramedics, who were now doing CPR. That's not a good sign, I thought. Patients that arrest in the field have less than a one-percent chance of survival.

By the time I was ready to go meet Harry after securing the helicopter, he was already on his way back with the patient and a couple of firefighters. I met them halfway, and as we trotted along, he gave me a brief version of what was happening.

"Twenty-four-year-old guy," he yelled over the noise of the rotors, "playing chicken with a train on his motorcycle. He's got a head injury, flail chest, and an amputated right leg. Initially he was breathing, but nothing now. The medics tried to get him intubated, but couldn't get it in. So we'll try and tube him in the helicopter en route. No sense in wasting any more time here."

I nodded, and helped the firefighters load the patient in the aircraft. After securing the back door, I did my last walkaround to check doors and cowlings. Then, as I was climbing in, I spotted a firefighter running toward the helicopter carrying a large plastic trash bag. Pete was already spooling up the engines in preparation for our departure. I held up a finger to signal Harry to wait a minute and ran back out. I briefly saw his expression of disapproval as I ran back—he was busy and needed help. I knew what he was thinking: his rookie partner had deserted him, prolonging our ground time, which we tried to keep to five minutes.

I ran down the hill toward the firefighter and he handed me the large plastic bag. "I think you'll need this," he yelled over the noise of the helicopter. I assumed he was handing me the patient's belongings. I nodded and ran back up the hill, where the high whine increased as Pete pushed the throttles forward, getting ready to lift off. As I was running, the bag, which probably weighed ten or fifteen pounds, was banging against my leg, and something sharp was poking me. Puzzled, I opened the bag and peered inside.

It was a leg. Neatly severed at mid-femur. With a tennis shoe on the foot. I was horrified, and held the bag far in front of me as I clumsily ran along.

As soon as I reached the helicopter door, I handed the bag to Harry and then jumped in, latched the door and belted in. I gave Pete the thumbs-up, indicating we were ready in the back. As soon as we cleared the landing zone, Harry, who was breathless from performing chest compressions and bagging by himself, keyed up the mike. "Where did you go?" he demanded, clearly perturbed. "We don't delay transport to collect patient belongings."

I had my hands full doing the chest compressions now, and I nodded towards the bag. "Well, it's not really belongings in the normal sense of the word," I yelled over the noise.

Harry reached over, opened the bag and peered in. "Jesus," he said. "You could have at least warned me."

I shrugged, and we got down to the business of getting the

patient intubated and pushing drugs to try and bring him back. Of course, there wasn't much left to get back. By the laws of gross tonnage, it seemed pretty clear that a train would win over a motorcycle every time, making this patient's planning seem somewhat shortsighted. Darwin was right.

By ten o'clock that night, we had finished all our paperwork and, despite my efforts to delay it, bedtime had arrived. Grabbing the nightclothes I had carefully chosen the previous night, I dashed into the bathroom. I put on a leotard, leggings, a T-shirt and a scrub suit, covering it all with a very large, ugly, stained terrycloth robe. After twenty minutes of brushing my teeth and scrubbing my face, I faced myself in the mirror. "Now Janice," I told myself firmly, "you're being ridiculous. This is a professional organization, and we conduct ourselves as professionals. Harry is not a midnight rapist. Now just march your bad old self out there and get into bed." Cautiously, I opened the door and peered out.

My worst fears were realized. Harry was leaning over his duffel bag, wearing nothing but his saggy BVDs. I whipped back into the bathroom, slamming the door behind me. Leaning against the wall, breathing heavily, I considered my options: either run screaming into the night, effectively ending my career as a flight nurse, or just deal with it. Surely Harry wasn't going to sleep in his underwear with a woman he barely knew? I leaned my head against the wall until my breathing slowed to normal.

After a few minutes, I stuck my head out the door again. Thankfully, Harry was now sitting up in bed, wearing a T-shirt, casually reading. "There you are," he said. "I was beginning to get worried about you. Everything all right?" He was obviously unaware of my discomfort.

"Uh, yeah, just fine," I answered, sidling past him, avoiding eye contact and diving into my bed, still swaddled in three layers of clothing. "I was just flossing." I turned away from him and picked up my book. "Pretty busy today, don't you think? Did I do OK? Boy, oh, boy, what a day. I can't wait to go home tomorrow and tell Mark all about this." I realized I was babbling and pulled my book closer. A strained silence filled the room.

About fifteen minutes later, I rolled over to shut off the light. Harry looked at me, obviously uncomfortable. "Um, Janice. I think I should tell you something. It's only fair."

Uh-oh, here it was. He was going to divulge some deep secret, and I barely knew him. Or maybe he was going to admit to some sexual deviance, or God only knows what. "What do you need to tell me?"

"Well, I have this problem."

"What kind of problem?" I asked, becoming more alarmed by the second. I was poised to scoop up my handbag and flee.

"Well, a problem with, uh, gas. You know, flatulence. Some people find it kind of distressing."

Relief flooded over me. He was worried because he had a little gas now and then? Didn't we all? "Oh, Harry, don't worry about it. I thought you were going to tell me you were some sort of twisted pervert."

He laughed, the tension broken. "No, it's not as simple as that. I don't think you understand. This isn't like regular gas. It's kind of, well, major gas."

"Believe me, you don't need to worry about that."

"I just wanted to warn you, that's all."

So this was the reason for the mysterious warning from JoAnn. I figured it was probably an ongoing CALSTAR joke. "Good night, Harry." I carefully placed my beeper next to the phone and arranged my boots and flight suit so I could quickly scramble into my clothes if we got that midnight call. Harry chuckled at my earnest efforts.

"You *are* a newbie," he said, stuffing his beeper into his

boots. "Aw, you'll figure it out soon enough." Shaking his head, Harry switched off the light.

I was determined only to doze, so I wouldn't sleep through an activation. Harry's breathing got slow and regular, then became a loud snore. "They didn't mention this," I thought to myself as I slowly settled into a deep sleep.

Suddenly the quiet was shattered by an explosion. I sat bolt upright trying to orient myself. Had a bomb gone off? Gunfire? Where was I? Where was Mark? Why was I in this strange bed? Then Harry's malady fully asserted itself. A foul cloud wafted over to my bed, causing me to sputter and cough. Harry, who had also been awakened by the sound, jumped straight up.

"We got a flight? Where are we going? Where are my boots?" He scanned the floor, searching wildly for his gear.

"Harry, calm down. We don't have a flight. You farted," I said, trying to hold my breath.

"My God, sure did," he replied, fluffing his bedcovers. "Boy, this is a bad one."

My eyes were watering, and I do believe the wallpaper was peeling. "Oh, Harry, please stop waving your sheets. You're only making it worse."

"Oops, sorry. Maybe I could open a window." He struggled out of bed and began pawing frantically through the heavy drapes to find an avenue for fresh air.

"Harry, the window doesn't open. We're on the ground floor of a hotel, remember? Just open the door and fan, OK? Jesus, you weren't kidding. I didn't thing human beings could create such a thing. It should be listed with Hazardous Materials."

After a while, the room aired out. My eyes had stopped watering, and we could both breathe again. "Harry, does this happen often?" I asked. "If this is an every-night occurrence, I might just take my chances in the pilot's room."

"Must have been those refried beans I had after dinner," he admitted. "Sorry. As long as I stay away from them and broccoli, I'm usually fine."

I sighed, turned over, and went peacefully to sleep. This was going to be a hell of a ride.

A Day in the Life

Iᴛ wasn't long before I started feeling comfortable with the CAL-STAR routine—if you can call it a routine.

We worked twenty-four-hour shifts, similar to firefighters. In the latter half of my time at CALSTAR I was based out of Concord, California, northeast of Oakland, at an airport known as Buchanan Field. We had various housing arrangements there over the years—converted offices, a hotel, a single trailer. Today the crew lives in comparative luxury, in a double-wide trailer with a separate room for everyone, but during my ten years at CALSTAR, I always had to share a bedroom with at least my shift partner. For a while all the crew slept in a large room, dormitory-style. That was sometimes difficult, because at least half of the pilots snored heavily. More than once I found myself sleeping in my car, that being the only peaceful spot I could find.

We lived together in these cramped quarters for an entire day, awaiting the call. We had a hot plate, an electric wok, a microwave, and a limited kitchen. We became pretty clever at finding ways to feed ourselves and pass the time.

A typical morning started with a crew change at 9:30. We would pull in, dragging our overnight bags and groceries, swapping hugs and hellos, gauging the off-going crew's condition. You could tell what kind of shift they had had by what they were doing—if it had been a quiet day, they'd be sitting around drinking coffee, doing some cleaning, finishing up some last-minute paperwork and packing their things to go home. If it had been a bad shift, they'd be sitting like zombies on the couch, or crouched over huge charts, malodorous, with rumpled hair and reddened eyes. Or sometimes they'd still be asleep, having got in only an hour before.

Usually both crews, and often the pilots too, would sit down for an official morning report, discuss memos from the office or needed supplies, arrange for the return or retrieval of equipment left at the hospital, and confirm any training drills we had for the day. We would then informally discuss the previous crew's flights and carry on the usual office gossip. Afterward, we headed out for morning preflight. For the nurses, this meant making sure all the equipment was present, in working condition, and clean. The pilots and the mechanic also did daily inspections.

Once preflight was done, we would head back into the office to complete the tedious paperwork: follow-up calls on all our patients every three days, reporting patient outcomes via letter to the agency that had requested our services, and then chart reviews for flights from the previous day. Each flight was reviewed by a peer, chief flight nurse, and our medical director. Interesting, unusual or difficult flights were flagged so we could review them later at staff meetings. Calls where we had done something invasive were also flagged for discussion in the monthly staff meetings, so we could learn from each other's experiences.

After the morning chores were done, we were free to do whatever we felt like—watch TV, read a book or do more paperwork. There is a lot of down time in any flight program, where you're just sitting and waiting for a call. Tim, one of the pilots, said it most succinctly: "They pay us to sit around quarters. The flying is for free." And it's true. Because of all the time we spent together in relative boredom, we all got to know one another well. I believe this is one of the secrets of CALSTAR's success—we knew each other so intimately that when we worked there was usually little discussion. Every move was carefully choreographed, and we learned each other's ways so well that we didn't need to talk.

When we got activated, we were in the air in five minutes, especially if it was a scene call. Usually at first we knew only the general area we were headed to, and maybe the type of incident. After we were airborne, we would get the exact location (this was before the advent of the global positioning system, or GPS), radio frequencies, and exactly what kind of call it was. If it was an interfacility call—transporting a patient from one hospital to another with a higher level of care or specialization—we might take a moment to make a phone call to clarify what was happening. More often than not, however, we would launch and work out the details en route.

Many times we were activated because the patient was in a remote location, or if the first responders—usually the fire department—felt there was a possibility of serious injuries. In the latter case, the paramedics sometimes arrived, assessed the patient, and decided that the person didn't require helicopter transport after all, and we would be canceled. These dry runs were routine, and they gave us a chance to get out of quarters and go for a helicopter ride. Of course we didn't like dry runs at 3:00 a.m., but that's all part of the job. We sometimes used the flying time for training, or maybe a bit of a scenic tour.

Flight nurses fly in one of two pre-determined roles—primary and secondary. The primary nurse is responsible for navigation to the scene and then managing patient care on the way home. The secondary nurse runs the radios, sets the helicopter up for the patient after landing, and then assists the primary in patient care. He or she is also responsible for aircraft safety on scene.

The number of calls per day varied dramatically. We were busiest in the summer, when the public was engaged in sports and outdoor activities that often involved alcohol or drugs. It wasn't unusual to do two or three flights per day, and my personal best was seven (others have beat that record). It is extremely taxing to do back-to-back flights, and when they stack up, it becomes exhausting, especially in the summer heat. I recall all too well dragging myself back into quarters at 6:00 a.m. with four charts to complete, weak from fatigue, almost willing to sell my soul for some sleep.

The winter months are different. There are fewer recreation-related accidents, and weather is often a problem. Around the beginning of December, a thick fog could descend. It would sometimes stick around for days and make it difficult to see the helicopter just fifty feet from the trailer. Of course, we weren't able to fly in those conditions. We had to go to work anyway and amuse ourselves as best we could, knowing full well we wouldn't be going anywhere for the duration. On those days, my husband referred to CALSTAR as the "nursing retirement home," and would regularly call to ask if we were developing bedsores from constant napping.

The crew would get grumpy as days passed without a flight. Those were difficult times—imagine being in the middle of a fog bank, confined to a small trailer with minimal amenities. Of course, fog could also be our friend. When a call came in at 4:00 a.m. and we couldn't even see the helicopter from the trailer, we could roll over peacefully knowing we weren't going anywhere.

One thing that made the job so interesting was that when I arrived at work each morning, I had no idea what might happen in the next twenty-four hours. Many of our flights were routine, but there were also ones that the pilots referred to as right-turn-only flights. The pilot sits in the right-hand seat, and the patient is on the left side of the helicopter. If the patient was truly a bloody mess, the pilots would joke that they would only make right turns so they wouldn't have to see the mangled human being. In reality, all the pilots had seen the worst, and many of them became quite sophisticated in their understanding of medical care, even to the point where they'd jokingly offer opinions on patient management. Sometimes they were right.

As I grew accustomed to life at quarters and got more flights under my belt, I learned the cardinal rules of the job. First off, a well-fed flight nurse is a happy flight nurse. We never really knew when the refrigerator lifeline might be severed for eight, ten, or twelve hours, so for the most part we were not very fussy eaters. When you're stuck for a full day with no access to outside food, a three-day-old pizza is a jealously guarded ace in the hole. Any visitor was invariably met with the question, "What did you bring us to eat?" If they had not brought edible offerings, we turned them away.

I quickly came to know my fellow crew members' food idiosyncrasies. One former colleague, for example, loved to barbecue week-old carp, creating an unbearable stench that added a certain flavor to anything else we grilled. Beth was a committed nibbler—I never saw her sit down to a full meal. Nancy was our junk-food queen, with a particular fondness for Hostess Snowballs. And Harry's food bag needed to be monitored carefully, for reasons already revealed. I inspected his groceries on arrival to ensure that no beans or bean by-products slipped in the door. Occasionally, he tried to sneak one by. For this, we had an emergency supply of Beano.

I got a hint about the second rule of flight nursing at my initial CALSTAR interview. The chief flight nurse had several queries regarding my bladder capacity, a pretty intimate subject to discuss with a complete stranger. However, I realized the questions were appropriate when confronted with a flight at 3:00 a.m. after consuming three cups of herbal tea before bedtime. After two hours of flying, my bladder was absolutely stretched to capacity, and every bounce of the helicopter made me wince in agony. There are no rest stops at 1500 feet, and I learned a very important lesson: go early, go often, go even if you think you don't need to.

The next flight nursing rule often works against the previous one: Never turn down a free drink. Especially in summer. Temperatures in the helicopter can easily surpass 110 degrees, and when combined with black long-sleeve Nomex flight suits and helmets, this can add up to misery. The air-conditioning system uses up precious power, so often it isn't used when the helicopter requires extra for takeoff and landing. The heat was not so bad when we flew along at 120 miles per hour and there was good air flow through the windows, but when the forward speed was reduced, the cabin quickly heated up. To prevent dehydration and hyperthermia, we carried bottles of Evian, slugging them down at every opportunity.

The last rule of flight nursing concerns sleep: Get it early, get it often, because you're never quite sure when you'll have an opportunity to catch a couple of Zs. It's inevitable that you will fly all day and night if you come to work tired. And the consequences for those bold enough to come to work after a frivolous night on the town are worse. The beeper gods take a particular delight in torturing those poor souls.

We developed a number of sleep rituals and superstitions. First of all, we made our beds upon arrival in the morning. Lord help the crew member who waited until ten o'clock at night to smooth the sheets onto the mattress. That virtually guaranteed a long night of flying, and wrestling with sheets at 6:00 a.m. after several intense calls is an ordeal only for the stout of heart. And since the nurses shared a room, the partner of such an ill-prepared crew member didn't appreciate the delay.

If there was an opportunity for an afternoon nap, I embraced it. Of course, this meant I sometimes wound up tossing and turning at 3:00 a.m., but that was preferable to doing back-to-back pediatric flights on only a few hours sleep.

Over the years, I developed a system for slotting patients into one of the three categories after the first thirty seconds of my assessment. The first and most common tier was where the patient fit into the category of "not hurt bad, everybody relax." These patients required the specialized services of a trauma center, but didn't have immediately life-threatening injuries. We could relax and just do our job.

The second and most frightening tier was, "I'm hurt real bad and if I don't get to a trauma center soon I'll die," otherwise known as SAS, or sick as shit. With these patients we had to make accurate and complete assessments quickly, and in order to buy them some time, we often had to perform extremely invasive procedures rapidly and precisely. These were the worst, the most challenging, but also the most interesting to manage. They were the reason I loved being a flight nurse.

The third was "this patient is doomed," where nothing we could do would change the inevitable outcome. While these patients made for a busy flight, we remained relatively calm because the only question was whether death would be imme-diate or delayed. We quietly referred to them as "dog lab" patients, since we could safely practise invasive procedures with them, thus preparing ourselves for future patients who might still be in the second tier.

This kind of triage took time to master, and on some of my early flights my assessment skills were still sorely lacking. On one occasion we were activated to Richmond for some sort of violent mayhem. Beth was my partner that day. As we landed, I grabbed the trauma bag and headed for the waiting ambulance.

A young man lay on the gurney, apparently unresponsive, meaning he would need an endotracheal tube to assist his breathing. I swallowed hard—this would be my very first field intubation. I came to the terrible realization that this poor man's life might well rest in my quavering, inexperienced hands. Fol-lowing my training, I dropped to the basics: airway, breathing, circulation. Yes, his airway was intact. But no, his breathing did not look normal to my inexpert eye. And did he have a Glasgow Coma Score of less than eight? I ran through the procedure to assess his level of consciousness.

"Hey!" I yelled at him. "Can you hear me?" Nothing.

Next was tactile stimulation. "Hey!" I yelled, shaking his shoulder. "Open your eyes." Nothing.

I moved on to painful stimulation. I put my knuckles on his chest and gave him a brisk sternal rub. Nothing again. All right, this was it. The moment had arrived. I was going to have to tube this patient, like it or not. I nervously grabbed the bag with the intubation equipment and unzipped it. Upside down. The entire contents of the bag fell to the floor with a crash.

At this moment, Beth appeared at the back door. She looked at me with some hesitation as I groped for the equipment, which was now spread over the floor of the ambulance. "What's going on?" she asked, looking carefully at our patient.

"This guy was assaulted, and he's not responding, so I'm gonna intubate him," I said. "I think."

"Why don't you try a nasal airway first to see if his nares are clear," she suggested.

I nodded, glad to delay that awful moment when I would be exposed as a fraud. I lubricated the tube and began to ease it into his left nostril. No response. For a second.

Without warning the patient opened his eyes and regarded me sullenly. "What the fuck you think you're doin', bitch?" he enunciated quite clearly. "Get that shit outta my nose."

"Oh, you're awake," I squeaked. "Uh, how do you feel?"

"I was fine till you stuck that motherfuckin' thing in my nose."

Later, as we flew home, I crouched down in my seat, feeling like an utter fool. How could I have been so far off base? This patient must have *chosen* not to cooperate, and he couldn't have had a serious head injury that warranted invasive procedures. How could I have been so stupid? And would I ever recognize the real thing when I saw it?

When we returned to base, I scurried off to restock the aircraft. Beth followed me into the supply closet, with a serious look on her face. "You, my dear, have just been witness to a common syndrome: JFA."

I racked my brain trying to figure out what she meant; I didn't want to appear ignorant. Junctional functional arrest? Jejuno-falsiform aporrhipsis?

"JFA," Beth explained. "Also known as a Jive Funk Attack. Couldn't be anything else. Very common in young males with no sense to know when somebody is trying to help them."

As a former Oakland paramedic, Beth knew that some of these guys, especially those in gangs, don't cooperate with anyone they associate with the police—and that includes fire, medics and flight nurses. They're too cool for that. Indeed, Beth knew that our "patient" was full of shit the moment she looked at him: He was pink, warm, dry, with normal respirations—all signs I failed to notice.

Would I ever be a real flight nurse?

Emotional Bunkers

The day had been a scorcher, with the thermometer registering over a hundred degrees at noon. At the CALSTAR base, I sat outside on the steps with Carrie and J.B., our pilot, enjoying the evening breeze. It had been a quiet shift so far, but we knew it didn't bode well for a full night's sleep. After the oppressively hot day, the evening would invite people outdoors all over the Bay Area, and tempers always seemed to flare with a heat wave, which usually meant business for CALSTAR. The "knife and gun club," as we called them, usually got busy around 10:00 p.m., and that hour was rapidly approaching.

I always enjoyed working with Carrie. At first glance, she seems to be the epitome of innocence. She is rather petite with large blue eyes and soft, curly blonde hair, and she comes off as rather soft-spoken and shy. When CALSTAR first hired her, we had a quick powwow before she showed up on her first day, and we were told to behave ourselves around her: No cussin', scratchin', or breaking wind. We were to behave professionally no matter what, for fear of driving this gentle creature away. That day was a horror. It started with a flight as soon as Carrie walked in the door, followed by three more in succession, and she stood up to it gracefully and tried as hard as she could to keep up with the pace. At 11:30 p.m. we finally sat down to eat and, of course, the phone rang immediately. Carrie let out a barrage of expletives that would make a sailor blush. She was just one of the gang thereafter.

"Should we start *The Fugitive?*" Carrie asked.

"We're sure to get a call right at the best part," J.B. replied, standing up and stretching. "But I've been wanting to see it. Might as well put it on." We trailed into quarters, and J.B. stuck the movie into the VCR. Carrie popped some microwave popcorn and we settled in.

Sure enough, just at the climax of the movie, the dispatch phone rang. At 11:45 p.m., that could only mean we were going for a helicopter ride. It was a scene call—we were to do a pickup of a shooting victim in Richmond and deliver him to John Muir Hospital.

Richmond is a ghetto north of Berkeley where poverty and violence are endemic. When CALSTAR first began flying into Richmond, we were faced with some hostility and danger, but over the years we developed a rapport with the Richmond Fire Department and were now just part of the scenery there. Many of the calls were the result of gang fights and drug deals gone awry, and violence was so commonplace that gang members were not considered initiated until they had had at least one ride with CALSTAR. Generally the victims had some sort of violent trauma—bullet wounds, stab wounds, and assaults—and some were repeat customers. Richmond calls were quick and exciting, but the appalling social ills eventually became depressing.

Dispatch advised us that we were to pick up a patient with a gunshot wound. The scene of the incident was not yet secure and we were to rendezvous with the ambulance at the helipad at Brookside, the local community hospital that didn't have the capacity for managing a major trauma patient.

Our flight time to Richmond would be about ten minutes, and there would be a return flight of eight or nine minutes to John Muir with the patient. Over the years we have been able to make this whole run—from skids-up to a completed chart in the rack—in less than ninety minutes. With luck, we might be able to get back to the movie by a little after 1:00 a.m.

As we lifted off into the tropical night, I felt that old exhilaration of flying. I smiled as J.B. banked the helicopter off to the west toward Richmond. The chattering of the radios, swapping traffic on the emergency frequencies, the noise and smell of the jet engines, all seemed reassuringly familiar. I keyed up the intercom. "J.B., do you need the waypoints for Brookside?"

"No," he replied. "I think the old girl could probably fly herself there without us." Indeed, we had made this same flight dozens of times. The routine, as grisly as it could be, was familiar and reassuring. Carrie and I began preparing everything to receive the patient—turning on the cardiac, blood pressure and oxygen-saturation monitors, and spiking an IV with tubing and flushing the air out to get it ready for our patient's arrival.

Our policy of landing at the Brookside helipad rather than at an unstable scene was the result of several unnerving situations. Since most of our calls to Richmond involved some sort of mayhem, there was nearly always quite a crowd around, and the police were not always successful in securing the land-ing zone. Whenever we landed on a scene we would invariably create a stir, and sometimes it almost turned into a riot. I remember pushing my way through an ugly-minded, uncon-trolled crowd one night and being really frightened. It was also dangerous for the people in the crowd if they got too close to the helicopter rotors.

Then there was the possibility that the guy with the gun was unapprehended, still in the crowd, and not keen on our ministrations to his intended victim. He might try to finish the job, either when we were on the ground or in the air. EMS folks get shot at fairly regularly, in fact, and although I don't know if a helicopter has ever been hit, it wasn't unreasonable. A helicopter can be shot out of the sky pretty easily, simply by hitting the tail rotor.

As we circled the Brookside helipad, I looked down and saw two fire engines and a police car. A group of men stood around drinking coffee. When the skids settled, J.B. keyed up the intercom.

"You're cleared out," he said. Grabbing the trauma bag, I headed off for the group. They were all talking and joking. They seemed relaxed, so I assumed our patient was not badly injured. I greeted the fire captain with a wave and a smile.

"How are you guys tonight?" he asked, taking a sip from his Styrofoam cup. "Hope we didn't interrupt anything."

"We were just at the best part of *The Fugitive*, but I guess that can wait. What have you dredged up for us?"

"Aw, just some guy who got shot," he said, shrugging.

"So I take it he's not too bad?"

"Actually, he's pretty much dead."

I didn't have time for more questions, as the ambulance was approaching with its lights flashing. As it pulled up in front of me, I saw a small rivulet of blood dripping out of the back doors. "This doesn't look good," I thought as I opened the door. A man was lying on the gurney, unresponsive, with blood gushing onto the floor of the ambulance from a gaping hole in his head. Along with the flow of blood, chunks of bone and brain tissue oozed off the backboard. One of the ambulance paramedics was at the head of the gurney trying to bag the patient, and it didn't appear to be going well. The second paramedic was trying to get an IV started. I glanced behind me. The firefighters and cops continued their lively discussion, ignoring the ambulance's arrival.

The first paramedic, Liz, whom I had met before, looked up and started telling me the story. "This is a twenty-year-old male with two gunshot wounds to the head—large-caliber gun at close range. He was initially hyperventilating and posturing, but is now somnolent with fixed and dilated pupils. There was a 500 cc blood loss on scene, and as you see it's still bleeding briskly. There was a lot of brain tissue on the ground where we found him. We're seeing agonal respirations, but have been unable to get him intubated." Agonal respirations look like a fish gasping for air—irregular, slow and ominous. They're a primitive reflex from deep within the brainstem and an indication that death is imminent.

As Liz was giving her report, I crawled up past the second paramedic to get to the head of the bed. My boots slipped in the pool of blood, and I nearly landed on my hip in the gruesome lake. As I got to the front of the gurney, I breathed a little sigh of relief—the wounds were all in the cranium, and the young man's facial structures appeared to be intact. I reached over and palpated his face and nose, which were stable. His eyes were partially open, with fixed and dilated pupils. The eyes were covered with a blue-tinged haze, indicating that he had, not surprisingly, lost his blink reflex. I pushed on his jaw, but it was clenched. This meant we had two options for securing his airway so we could get oxygen into him. One was to put in a nasotracheal tube, but this is a blind technique and there's always the possibility of "tubing the goose"—that is, putting the tube down his esophagus instead of his trachea. The other option was to intubate him orally, but since his jaw was clenched, we would have to do a rapid sequence induction (RSI) and paralyze him first. He didn't yet have an IV established to give him the necessary drugs, so we would have spent more time on the ground trying to do that. And clearly this man wasn't going to get any better lying in an ambulance.

I considered the options. If the paramedics had already had trouble getting the tube in, he probably didn't have an easy airway. In addition, after multiple intubation attempts, the airway was probably pretty beat up and bloody, making my subsequent efforts more difficult. I thought a nasotracheal tube might work out better and, if I couldn't get it in, we would do an RSI in the helicopter en route to John Muir.

Carrie arrived at the back of the ambulance and stood for a minute surveying the carnage. "What a mess," she commented as she climbed into the back.

I gave her a brief report, relaying my plan for a nasal tube. She nodded as she helped me set up my equipment. "Facial bones intact?" she asked. "Don't want this tube to head north and end up in his midbrain."

"Yeah, looks like most of the trauma is in the cranium itself. He's got only agonal respirations, but at least he's breathing enough to help guide the tube in." I squirted Neo Synephrine up our patient's nose, pulled out a 7.5 endotracheal tube and covered it in numbing lidocaine jelly. Gently I inserted it into his nose. "Please go in, please go in," I muttered as I passed it through the nasal turbinates and watched for a mist as he exhaled. With each breath, I gently advanced it further until he coughed slightly, and a little blood squirted out of the end of the tube. We were in. I inflated the balloon and murmured a quiet prayer of thanks to the intubation gods. Carrie handed me an $ETCO_2$ monitor, which confirmed that we were in the right spot. Liz whipped out a stethoscope and listened to the chest for breath sounds as I bagged.

As Liz handed me the tape to secure the tube, the second medic hit a vein and got the IV hooked up and secured. While Carrie and the medics quickly finished packaging the patient—that is, immobilizing him on the backboard—I was able to suction out our patient's airway. We were set to go.

During all of this, I was vaguely aware of loud laughter outside the ambulance. The group of firefighters and cops had grown, and there were now about fifteen people milling around outside cracking jokes. Liz stuck her head out of the ambulance and asked for four people to load the gurney onto the helicopter. No one heard her, and they continued to talk loudly. She became exasperated.

"Do you guys think you can break away from your fun for a minute and help us get the goddamn patient loaded?" she yelled over the noise.

Several of the firefighters turned, looking surprised, and a couple of them grabbed the end of the gurney as we slid it out of the ambulance. The rest of the group turned back to their discussion.

"Carrie," I said, "take over the airway while I go get the aircraft set up, OK?" She nodded, and took over bagging. I clambered out of the back of the ambulance and walked down to the helipad. I threw the trauma bag over the seat of the helicopter and turned on the monitors, expecting the crew to be there to load the patient. Instead, they were still at the back of the ambulance. Liz appeared to be yelling at one of the cops, and she was shaking her fist in his face. He had his hands on his hips and was yelling back at her. "What the hell?" I wondered aloud.

At that point, Carrie gently took Liz's shoulder, and pulled her away from the cop, at the same time pushing the patient toward the helicopter. I could see Liz get in one last shot at the cop as they wheeled the gurney down to the heliport ramp. Together we loaded our unfortunate patient into the helicopter and in a moment lifted off into the night. I glanced at my watch. We had been on the ground for twelve minutes.

As soon as we were airborne, we started hooking our patient up to the monitors. His initial blood pressure was 240/160, coupled with a heart rate of 160. I sat back for a minute, trying to figure out what might be happening with this man. High blood pressure with a head injury pointed to a clinical syndrome known as herniation. After a head injury, the brain swells, just like an ankle after it's sprained. Since the brain is enclosed in a bony compartment that does not expand with the swelling, the pressure keeps increasing. The tissue literally gets squeezed out through the only outlet available, the foramen magnum, which is the hole at the base of the skull where the spinal cord emerges. As one would imagine, this is not a good thing. Herniation is usually accompanied by a slow heart rate and an irregular breathing pattern. The usual intervention is to drill several holes in the skull, known as burr holes, to try and relieve some of the pressure. In this case, however, it didn't add up. The patient's heart rate was too high, and he already had two huge holes in his cranium from the gunshot wound, which continued to ooze blood and gray matter. And he still had only agonal respirations.

No, this didn't make sense. Maybe it was a problem with

the monitors, or maybe the vibration of the helicopter had caused the abnormal reading. I reached over and took another blood pressure. This was much more what I expected—80/30, which reflected the enormous blood loss he had suffered. Carrie looked at the monitor, nodded, and started pushing the fluids to replace what he had lost. With the bag, I hyperventilated our patient to blow off the CO_2 he had undoubtedly accumulated before being intubated. This maneuver also helped to decrease the brain swelling by constricting the blood vessels between the brain and the skull.

All of this activity was futile. With this injury, the patient had no hope of meaningful survival, even though his heart was still beating. This man was going to die; the only question was when. The best we could hope for was stabilization until he could be evaluated for organ donation. Patients with gunshot wounds to the head are perfect organ donors. Generally they are young men in perfect health with a single exception: They no longer have a functional brain.

As we arrived in the trauma room at John Muir, we moved the patient off the helicopter's backboard onto the hospital's gurney. A large chunk of gray matter slid off our litter and splattered onto the floor. The trauma surgeon regarded this impassively and returned to his evaluation.

A quiet descended over the room as the team started their workup. None of the usual frantic activity of a trauma room was apparent; everyone knew what the outcome of this case would be. In the bright lights of the room, I now saw the telltale track marks in the man's veins, indicating IV drug use. That meant he would probably be a lousy candidate for organ harvest.

Carrie and I gathered up our equipment and headed for the workroom to start the distasteful task of paperwork. As soon as we were out of earshot of the staff, I turned to Carrie. "What was going on back there at the helipad? It looked like Liz and that cop were about to get into a fistfight."

Carrie stretched and yawned. "She got upset because of their attitudes. She thought she was trying to save somebody's life, and they were all acting like they were at the beach. I guess she took it personally."

I understood Liz's hostility. She was trying to do her job, which in this case was saving another human being's life, and she felt the cops' behavior didn't reflect the gravity of the situation. But I could see the cops' side, too. They saw this carnage first-hand—beatings, shootings, stabbings, drug overdoses. While we at CALSTAR usually only saw the ones that were alive, if only barely, they witnessed man's inhumanity to man over and over, day after day. In order to cope with this brutality, they learned to build a thick insulating shell around themselves. Even the most macho of men must go home and cry alone in a closet after they've seen a murdered toddler or heard a burn victim scream-ing in agony. Building an enormous emotional bunker is the only way they can survive.

Our patient died later that night. He was found to be HIV-positive, decisively precluding him from organ donation. The shooting turned out to be over a quarter gram of crack. This man was someone's son, brother, husband, friend. And yet I found myself surprisingly unmoved. I simply found the whole incident a stupid waste of a life. I guess I've built a bit of an emotional bunker myself.

One of the things we have to do as caregivers, ironically, is learn to care for ourselves. That's often difficult—after a time, nurses don't recognize their own needs, even immediate ones. There are times, however, when we have to withdraw from the work after a particularly painful call.

The first time this happened to me I never opened my trauma bag. There was no gore, no haunting screams—there wasn't even a body. And yet it was one of the worst calls I ever went on.

It was a warm summer afternoon, and CALSTAR was activated to Lake Del Valle, above the Livermore Valley. The dispatcher informed us we were going after a "drowning victim, UTL," or unable to locate. None of us was terribly concerned. With many UTL calls, the victim has merely wandered off to the snack bar or is taking a nap somewhere. We usually got canceled before we even reached the scene.

With Carl at the controls, we flew toward Del Valle, getting the details of the incident over the radio. A middle-aged couple had taken their small fishing boat out on the lake. While they were twenty yards off shore in fifteen feet of water, the husband had fallen overboard and not come back up. The wife had jumped in the water to try and grab him, then was unable to climb back into the boat. Ranger units spotted her and pulled her and the boat back to shore. The husband had still not been found. Several bystanders and rangers were now in the water trying to locate him.

This changed the story completely. If there were witnesses, this was probably a real drowning after all. The clinical implications changed as well. The man was thought to have gone down forty-five minutes ago. If that was true, it would be difficult to get anything back if they could find him. Patients pulled from the water often get full-court-press resuscitation, as the cold may help to preserve cardiac and neurological function. Only problem was, those magnificent saves were usually in water that was hovering around freezing. Lake Del Valle's temperature was probably sixty-five to seventy degrees, making the preserving hypothermia a moot point at best.

As we approached the lake, Carl got instructions to land

on a nearby lawn, in hopes the body would be recovered soon after we touched down. On the ground, we could see a large group of people huddled on the beach watching the rescue efforts. There were about six people in the water around an anchored Zodiac ranger skiff. This was not a high-tech rescue effort. The dive team had been mustered, but would not be there for some time. Meanwhile, the rangers and several bystanders were merely holding their breath, diving down and feeling around in the murky water, then popping back up to the surface, gulping air. Although this was not very efficient, there was no other alternative until the dive team arrived. Time was running out.

Nancy, who was flying primary, grabbed the bag and headed over to the incident commander's group. They were preparing to launch another small boat and they wanted Nancy to go with them so she could begin rendering care as soon as they pulled the victim out of the water. I stayed back to provide security until Carl could shut down the helicopter. The rangers had cordoned off the beach, and a large crowd had gathered to watch. Occasionally a child would cry, but otherwise a relative hush lay over the scene as the high whine of the helicopter died out.

A woman stood alone on the beach, intently watching every move of the activity, oblivious of the silent crowd behind her. I knew this must be the wife. Part of me shrank back—after all, what is there to say when you are watching a team drag the bottom of a lake for your husband's body?

Tentatively I approached her and placed my hand on her shoulder. "Hi," I said. "I'm Janice, one of the helicopter nurses. Can I get you anything?"

She turned away from the lake for just a second and looked at me through teary eyes. "No," she said tersely. "God damn it, they're looking in the wrong place."

"Where should they be looking?" I asked.

"Over to the left," she said dully. "They need to be over to the left. I told them that, but nobody would listen."

"I'll relay that to them," I said, reaching for my portable radio. "Nancy, this is Janice. I'm with his wife. She says you people need to be over to the left by about ten feet or so. You're looking in the wrong place."

"Copy that," she replied from the boat. "Will advise." There was a pause while Nancy relayed the message to the dive team. "They're having a hard time because the water is so murky down there. The divers have exhausted the area to our left, and think the current may have moved him down to where they're looking now."

I turned back to the woman. "They think the current might have washed him farther south. That's why they're looking there. They couldn't find him farther up to the left, OK?" She nodded, and continued to stare. "What is your name?"

"Jenny," she said. I noticed for the first time she was soaking wet and shivering violently. The afternoon breeze was freshening, and she was wearing the same clothes as when she had jumped into the lake. Gently, I touched her shoulder.

"Jenny, listen. You're shivering. Do you have any dry clothes we can get you into? We need to get you dried off."

She roughly brushed my hand off her shoulder. "Will you leave me alone?" she shouted. "Can't you see that wet clothes don't mean anything? I don't care. Now leave me alone." She turned away from me, tears flowing down her cheeks.

She was right. At that moment in her life, the only thing that mattered were those people out there trying to pull her husband out of the water. Everything else was incidental, unimportant. I realized I had been using the wrong approach. I walked over to the lawn and grabbed a beach chair, then found a blanket. Carrying them back to the beach, I spoke to her quietly. "Jenny, here, why don't you at least sit down and put this blanket around you. You're going to get sick being in the wind like this."

She glared at me for a moment, then obediently sat down. I tucked the blanket around her, and sat down next to her, staying quiet. She continued to watch intently, crying quietly. The minutes ticked by. About ten minutes later, I tried again.

"Jenny, can you tell me what happened?" I asked.

She didn't take her eyes off the water. "Me and my husband George were out there fishing. He started complaining of pressure in his chest, so we decided we better get in and go for help. But the engine quit. He was standing at the back of the boat, trying to crank the engine, even though I told him I'd do it. Then I saw him kind of just sink to his knees, and then go headfirst overboard. I tried to grab him but he was too heavy and he slipped out of my hands. He just sank, like he wasn't even trying to swim. He wasn't even trying. I lost my grip, and he just sank away from me. Oh, God, if I could have only hung onto him. I jumped into the water after him, but he was gone. Then I couldn't get back into the boat. If I could have only hung onto him, he'd be OK. It's all my fault." She collapsed into great heaving sobs. "It's all my fault," she repeated, choking.

I put my arms around her. "Jenny, you couldn't possibly have pulled him back into the boat. He was too heavy. You did everything you could. You actually did everything right. If you hadn't gone for help right away, all these people wouldn't be looking for him. Believe me, this is not your fault."

After listening to her story, it sounded like George had probably had a heart attack and then a cardiac arrest before falling into the water, making a resuscitation now even more unlikely. I wasn't about to share this information with her. I sat there and rocked her as she continued to cry.

By now the dive team had arrived and was in the water,

feeling their way across the muddy bottom with their hands. The rangers continued to dive, feel around, surface for air, then go down again. It was clear that everyone was running out of hope. The sun was getting ready to set, and the temperature dropped another ten degrees. Jenny was starting to shiver again.

"Jenny, listen. Give me your car keys, and I'll go to your car and get you some dry clothes. You can stay right here and watch. I'll bring them back to you, OK? You're not doing yourself any favors sitting in these damp clothes."

She nodded and rummaged through her purse. "Oh shit," she said. "George has the car keys in his pocket. I can't even get into the car. What am I supposed to do now?"

She wasn't thinking this far ahead, but sooner or later she would need to get home. And she could use family or friends there for support. I could call them and have them come up and meet us here with a change of clothes and extra keys to the car. In the meantime, she really needed some dry clothes. I had no extras, but maybe someone in the crowd did. "Stay here, Jenny," I said. "I'll be right back."

Walking to the edge of the beach where the crowd still watched silently, I called out, "Does anybody have any extra dry clothes? This lady is soaking wet, and we need to get her dried off. I need a sweatshirt and pants if anybody has any." Almost every person started rummaging through their bags. A Hispanic man approached me, clutching a sweatsuit and a blanket.

"Will this help?" he asked in broken English. "It's all I have."

"Thanks," I said. "Write down your address and I'll try to have these returned to you, OK?"

He waved me off. "Don't worry about it," he said, "it is not worth it."

"Thanks so much," I said, and ran back down to the beach. Jenny had not moved.

"Jenny," I said gently, "we got some dry clothes for you. Why don't we go over to the restroom and get you changed. We should probably call somebody to come over with another set of car keys to get you home, too, OK?"

She looked back at the lake, then at me. "OK," she said, slowly getting out of the chair. We walked slowly toward the restroom. Occasionally she would pause, turn back, and watch the lake. Then she stopped and turned to me with a steady stare. "He's dead, isn't he?" she asked quietly.

For a moment, I wasn't sure what to say. I didn't want to take away her last shred of hope. But I couldn't lie. "Yes, Jenny, I think he is," I said softly.

"I knew that. I just needed to hear it." She started walking quickly for the bathroom, where I helped her change clothes. We didn't speak. I then led her outside to the pay phone and handed her some change. I asked if she wanted me to stay while she called her family, but she shook her head.

"I need to call our son. I'd like to do this alone."

"Whatever you wish," I said. "I'll be right over here if you want me."

We waited and watched at the water's edge for another hour, but the divers were unable to locate the body. Night was rapidly approaching, and Carl was overdue to go home. As much as we didn't want to admit it, there was no point in our participation any longer. If they did find the man, he couldn't be anything but dead by this time. We needed to get back in service and do a crew change. Despite this, I couldn't leave Jenny by herself. Not, at least, until her son showed up. I thought about how she must feel, how I would feel if, by some horrible chance, that was Mark in the cool murky water. George was gone and Jenny, in a sense, became our patient.

Jenny's son showed up a half-hour later. As soon as she

saw him, she collapsed into his arms, sobbing. We packed up our gear, forgotten, and prepared to head home. I watched them for a moment, then gently touched her shoulder. "Jenny, we have to go now. You'll be OK. I want you to remember you did everything you could. There was nothing you could do to change this, OK?"

She nodded and briefly hugged me. "Thanks," was all she said.

I have seen grief many times in my career, but this was the first call where I had any time to connect with a family member so intensely. It's not an easy thing to sit with someone who has just lost her husband, much less be the one to break the news. Besides, usually we were *doing* something, which would give us some focus; to simply sit and wait was far more difficult. Reflecting on this, I was feeling pretty beat up as we landed back at CALSTAR quarters.

When I got inside there was a brief message from Mark: "Call me at home."

When Mark answered the phone, I could tell something was wrong. "Honey, I'm sorry," he said. "Your mom called about an hour ago. Your Aunt Adrienne died today." She had been ill for over a month, but was not expected to die. This news put me over the edge. I walked out, handed the keys and beeper to Nancy and left. I was done for the day.

The Amazing Jim

Having participated in hundreds of flights, many of them unremarkable, there remains one that I will never forget. It's memorable not only because of its outcome, but because it probably logs in as the world's longest scene call.

Harry and I were working that night, with Vicki as our pilot. Vicki is small, slender blonde who shrieks tomboy. By the time she was hired at CALSTAR, everyone seemed to know her and the guys had all tried to get some time with her. Whenever she flew, the towers would want to chat and nearby aircraft would always ask us to come up on a non-official frequency to flirt with her. She rarely went out with them.

When we got the call, it was Elise on the phone from dispatch. "Hi, Janice. There's been a big rig accident in southern Santa Clara County and they've requested a helicopter. Highway 152 south of Gilroy. I'll contact you en route with the coordinates. About twenty-minute ETA from liftoff?"

"That would be about right. Catch you in a few minutes on the air."

Harry and I sprinted off to the helicopter, where Vicki was already cranking up. We climbed aboard, belted in, and were off into the night sky. I immediately keyed up the radio to get the details from dispatch.

"CALSTAR One," said Elise, "these are two trucks that hit head-on. Your patient is still being extricated. You will be talking to CDF Engine 5102 on fire white, 154.280. San Jose Medical Center is open and accepting."

"Good copy for CALSTAR One."

As we proceeded down the valley, we peered over the darkened landscape, looking for emergency beacons. "Boy," Harry said. "152 is only two lanes there, and if they really went head to head, this could be a mess. I wonder which truck won?"

"Obviously not the guy we're going for," Vicki concluded.

The scene was not hard to find. The Santa Clara Valley is mostly flat, and the gathering of emergency vehicles in a relatively rural area is pretty easy to spot, especially at night. I keyed up the radio again.

"Engine 5102, this is CALSTAR. We have you in sight. We should be overhead in two to three minutes. We will be approaching from the north, and we have just activated our Night Sun. Do you have a visual on us?"

It's hard to imagine being unable to spot a helicopter with a Night Sun—it can light up the ground brighter than day. Harry stood in front of it one time when they were testing it, and in less than thirty seconds it melted his pants and burned him.

"That's affirm," the firefighter replied. "You will be landing in a field just to the east of the accident. There are wires on the east side of the road, but otherwise no obstructions. The field is plowed dirt, and we have watered it down for you."

"Copy that. Be overhead in a few," I replied.

There was little moonlight and as we orbited the scene, checking out the landing zone, we were impressed with the spectacle on the ground. There were indeed two double tanker trucks, but both were now unrecognizable, and the wreckage was spread over a hundred yards. One of the trailers was obviously leaking some sort of white fluid, which covered the roadway. I prayed this wasn't some exotic chemical, making this a hazardous materials spill—a total nightmare. "Uh, Engine 5102. We see fluid leaking from one of the trailers. Have you identified the cargo of this vehicle?"

"CALSTAR One, we have identified the cargo as milk." All three of us breathed a small sigh of relief, and we circled the scene one more time to identify all the potential hazards, then turned short final. As soon as we were on the ground, Harry snatched the scene bag and headed off to the crowd of firefighters surrounding one of the trucks. As the ambulance arrived, I recognized the paramedics, Jamie and Tom.

"Jamie," I yelled over the noise of the helicopter. "What's going on with this guy? Do you know how much longer it will be before they can extricate him?"

Jamie shook his head. "From the looks of it, we're going to be here a while. All we have access to is his head and part of one arm. The whole truck is more or less on top of him. And I mean the *whole* truck. The engine is perched on top of what used to be the passenger compartment, which is crushed in around him."

"Should I tell Vicki to shut down the helicopter?"

"Yeah. It's going to be at least an hour, probably more." I nodded and headed back to the running helicopter.

"We can shut down," I yelled, motioning with my hand.

"It's gonna be at least another hour." Vicki nodded and pulled back the controls. As the screaming of the jet engines died out, the noise of the Jaws of Life and the fire department's diesel compressor took over. Ducking under the still-moving rotors, I trotted over to the scene to help Harry.

When I got closer, I saw Jamie had not been exaggerating. The firefighters were huddled around a twisted heap of unrecognizable metal over twenty feet tall. Jagged chunks of metal were strewn everywhere. Harry was now hanging upside down through the rear window of the cab while the firefighters were attempting to cut through the metal. Every time they cut something apart, the wreck would collapse in another spot.

I approached the incident commander. "Can I go talk to my partner?" I asked. "He may need some help."

"Yeah, just go around to the other side so you're not in the way."

I scurried around the corner, and crawled over the wreck behind Harry. "Yo, Harry, what can I do to help?" I asked, looking over his shoulder into the cab. Our patient was lying on his left side, with only his head, neck, left shoulder and left arm visible. Everything else was buried in the twisted metal. He appeared to be awake, but only marginally so. The paramedics had placed a cervical collar on him, but were unable to access any more of his body. Harry craned his neck toward me.

"Get the airway kit out for me," he said. "He's nodding yes and no, but can't talk because he's so short of breath. I think his chest wall is pretty tightly wedged in there, so he's gotta have a thoracic injury. I want to nasally intubate him now before his respiratory status gets any worse."

I nodded and crawled out feet first. I returned with the intubation equipment and a fresh tank of oxygen. As I crawled back into the wreckage, dragging the equipment behind me, I felt a sharp pain in my thigh. I looked down and realized I had caught my pants on a jagged piece of exposed metal, which had ripped into my flight suit and cut my thigh. "Damn," I muttered, "now I gotta get a tetanus shot." I pushed the bag toward Harry, then handed in the fresh bottle of oxygen. He carefully handed out the exhausted tank. "Hey, can you guys out there hear me?" he yelled to the firefighters over the noise.

"Hold up," I heard a firefighter yell. The din of the compressor stopped temporarily.

Harry yelled out. "Listen. I'm going to intubate this guy, so can you give me about three minutes? I need to be able to listen for breath sounds and confirm placement. We got oxygen tanks in here, so let me know if you're generating any sparks. I don't want to give this truck any reason to catch fire. I'm pretty well wedged in here."

The incident commander peered into the compartment. "No problem. Let us know when we can crank up again. The oxygen tank is OK for now, but the fuel tank is partially ruptured. We're pumping out the rest of the diesel in the tank now."

Harry nodded, then turned back to the patient. "Sir, can you hear me? Just nod yes if you can." The patient nodded imperceptibly. "Great. Listen. We're gonna get you out, but it's going to take a while. You were in an accident, and that's what got you pinned in here. Try not to move your head. Are you having trouble breathing?" Our patient mouthed yes. "OK, great, you can understand me. Listen, I have to put a tube down in your windpipe. It may be uncomfortable going in, but it will make it easier to breathe, OK?" Harry introduced the tube into the patient's nose and advanced it with each breath. Suddenly, the patient began to cough, and Harry began to help his respirations with the bag. After a few minutes his breathing slowed and our patient relaxed. Harry reached over and listened to his chest, what was visible anyway, and smiled. "All right, we have him tubed," he yelled. "Hand me up a blanket before you start again so we don't get showered with glass." Someone handed a blanket up to me, and I passed it to Harry and started to back out.

"Harry, I'll be right outside. Let me know if you need anything, or if you need to rest, and I'll spell you for a while." The sound of ripping metal obscured his answer. I stood outside with the medics, feeling totally helpless. The priority was simply to free this man, and there was nothing I could do to help. I could only get out of the way and let them do their job.

Twenty minutes of trying to pry through the metal made it obvious the extrication team wasn't getting anywhere. They had only been able to release the left arm, but the rest of his body continued to be hopelessly buried under the metal. One of the paramedics had crawled in to help Harry start an IV in the arm they had recently released, but there was still nothing the medical team could do.

The fire department started a new approach. Each time they pried open a section, they started using expanding hydraulic power bars to prevent it from re-collapsing. This meant they needed to call for aid from neighboring fire departments. One by one, new fire trucks began to arrive, carrying equipment. Soon fifteen fire engines were parked around the vicinity, with everyone's attention focused on freeing one man.

After standing around feeling useless for half an hour, I realized my leg was oozing a little blood, and I still had some paperwork to do from a previous patient. I leaned into the cab again. "Harry, would it be OK if I went into the ambulance and did my chart from our last call? I can't get in there to help you, and I cut my leg on some metal, so I need to get it cleaned up. Jamie and Tom can come get me if you need anything."

"Sure. But could you tell them to get me another O_2 tank?

I'm down to less than 250 here." I yelled to Jamie, who scurried off to get a new tank.

As I walked down the dark road toward the helicopter, I stumbled and almost fell over a solid piece of metal. I looked down, and saw a circular piece of metal about a foot in diameter, deeply imbedded in the asphalt. "What the hell?" I wondered aloud. A firefighter heard me as he was walking by, and shined his flashlight on the object wedged in the road.

"My God," he said. "Do you have any idea what that is?"

I shook my head. "A big chunk of metal is the best I can come up with."

"It's a clutch plate from the truck. That sucker must weigh seventy pounds." We looked back toward the accident, which was a good hundred feet from us. It must have flown off the truck during the impact and wedged itself into the pavement. Pretty impressive.

"Do you know what happened?" I asked.

"Yeah, I talked to the other driver before they took him to the hospital. He wasn't hurt too badly. A mule from the field over there wandered out into the road, and he swerved to try and avoid him. Unfortunately, there was another tanker truck right there, and they hit head on. Thank God neither one of them was hauling any hazardous materials. Then we'd really be up the creek."

"So how did the mule do in all of this?"

The firefighter swung his flashlight over to the ditch beside the road. The mule was lying on its back with all four legs straight up in the air.

When I got to the aircraft I found Vicki standing in the field, talking with the man who owned this ranch. I briefed her on the situation, grabbed the chart, and headed back toward the wreck. As I was jumping over the ditch by the road, I felt my foot sink into something squishy. I looked down, thinking I had stomped on a cow patty. To my horror, it was a very neat pile of entrails—the entrails of that unfortunate mule. He had been hit hard enough to jar the organs out of his body, and they had landed in a neat pile some twenty feet away. The visceral membrane was still intact, making it a tidy little sack of guts. I felt my stomach turn.

As I got back to the accident scene, Harry was standing outside and Tom's feet were sticking out of the back of the cab. I could see no real improvement in the extrication. Harry's hands had gotten tired from bagging, so the medical crew had started rotating inside for relief. There was still nothing I could do, so I headed off to the ambulance to start my chart. I glanced at my watch. It was now 2:45 a.m., and we were no closer to freeing our patient than three hours before. I turned my attention to the laceration on my thigh and gingerly dabbed the wound with Betadine, wincing in pain. After carefully cleaning it, I taped a four-by-four dressing over the top.

An hour later, I had all the paperwork complete and I climbed out of the ambulance, stiff and sore. No, they still weren't any closer to getting our patient out. The problem remained the same: Every time they cut something apart, the weight of the huge diesel engine would collapse the metal somewhere else. They were now using pneumatic pillows in addition to the power bars to support the structure, but that still wasn't enough. And to make matters worse, all of their efforts had destabilized the huge weight of the engine, and the whole thing threatened to topple and crush anyone inside or near the cab.

Harry, Jamie and Tom were all starting to tire from the hours of bagging this man. I crawled into the cab for my turn. I gently helped the patient breathe with the bag and pulled the blanket over us. I could see "Jim" embroidered on his shirt. His face was covered with dried blood.

"Is your name Jim?" I asked, and he nodded. "Hi Jim. I'm Janice. I'm one of the helicopter nurses, and I'm going to stay with you for a little while. You're probably pretty scared about now, huh?" Again, a little nod. "I can understand that. The fire-fighters are trying to get you out, but you're pretty well wedged in here. But they'll get you out. Are you having a lot of pain?" I asked, stroking his cheek. Jim nodded slightly. He followed my every move with his eyes. I reached down to feel his radial pulse, which was strong but rapid, and turned up his IV, which was getting low. "Hey you guys, can you get me another IV? This one is almost out." I glanced over to the portable oxygen tank, which was also nearly empty. "And an O_2 tank, too," I yelled over my shoulder. "Hey Harry, what do you think about giving him some morphine? He's got a blood pressure, and we're going to be here for a while."

"The trauma surgeon may not like it, but let's try to titrate a little in at a time," he said, and fetched an IV, an oxygen tank and a syringe with morphine.

"One more thing," I yelled. "Can somebody hand me a couple of damp four-by-fours? His face is covered in blood." I stuck my hand out, and was handed a stack of four-by-four dressings and a bottle of sterile saline.

I spiked the new IV, switched the tanks, and then gave Jim small amounts of morphine until his face relaxed a bit. Pulling the blanket over both of us, I gently washed the blood off his face, and then cradled his head in the crook of my arm, quietly talking to him about nothing in particular. I simply wanted him to know another human being was there with him. The whole scene was almost surreal; flashing red lights and the bright white truck lights were filtered through the blanket, muting them. Occasionally we were showered with glass, but under the blanket we were warm and protected.

It was now 4:30 a.m. They had been able to get down to his chest, but no farther. His right arm had been freed, but was badly fractured in several places, and his chest was badly bruised with some unstable rib fractures. We still couldn't get to his back. Unfortunately, when they released his chest, his level of consciousness had deteriorated but in a way that was merciful. He was still obviously terrified and, despite the morphine, in a great deal of pain. His blood pressure was also starting to drop.

Jim's time was running out. The incident commander and the firefighters realized it was useless to continue, and we had to make a move. The new plan was risky, but no one could come up with a better one. The idea was to lasso the engine with chains, and a tow truck with a large crane would pull it up, allowing us to slip Jim out from underneath. The problem was that there was a very real chance the engine could come loose from the cradle of chains and fall onto Jim. But, in a way, it really didn't matter. We already knew he had head, chest, and abdominal trauma. We assumed his pelvis was broken and that he had major lower extremity trauma. If we didn't get him out soon, he would die trapped inside the wreckage.

The incident commander ordered us out of the cab. They hooked up the winch and started slowly pulling, lifting the engine. There was a loud popping and scraping from the twisted metal, but it was moving. When it had been lifted two feet, the firefighters were able to open the side door, which had been pinned against the pavement. We slid in a backboard and started to pull on his torso, but after getting his hips and thighs disentangled we hit a snag. Harry and I crouched in the dirt, holding Jim's spine in alignment. One of the firefighters reached in and found the problem: Jim's right foot was twisted around the brake pedal, and it was wedged in tight. They threaded in the Jaws of Life—a hydraulic tool that looks like a pair of scissors on steroids—and tried to pry it off, but it was firmly planted under the demolished dashboard. Harry turned to the medics, who were holding Jim's torso.

"Does he have any pulses?"

Jamie reached over to get a femoral pulse. "Just barely," he said. "We don't have much time."

I could see Harry's mind racing. "I hate to even think of this," he said. "But we're going to have to amputate his foot unless anybody else has any ideas. He's going to die soon." We aren't trained or qualified to perform such a task. Sure, it's a relatively easy thing to do, and Jim had no perfusion to that foot, so the bleeding would be minimal. And he probably was going to lose the foot anyway. In a last-ditch effort, Harry reached in and pulled as hard as he could, while the fireman pushed with the jaws of the tool.

Suddenly he came free. Relieved, we pulled him out onto the backboard, face down, then put another backboard on top and turned him over. The injuries we hadn't been able to see were worse than we thought. He had several large abrasions and bruising over his chest and back with unstable rib fractures. His pelvis was mushy, indicating a bad fracture. His abdomen was tense and distended. Both femurs were fractured, and his right ankle had an open angulated fracture. We all feverishly started applying the backboard straps to secure him, then headed for the helicopter as fast as we could. As we were headed across the field, I saw a huge pile of oxygen tanks. "What are all of those?" I asked a nearby firefighter.

"That's all the oxygen we burned while we were sitting here. Your patient used up every O_2 tank in the South Valley, and we've been shuttling O_2 from San Jose for the past two hours. Last count we used twenty-one tanks."

We lifted off from the scene, heading for San Jose Hospital. En route we started a third IV and feverishly poured in fluids. When we arrived, we hit the ER at a dead run. Jim had not regained consciousness and his blood pressure was barely palpable. The trauma team descended on him as we backed out the door.

I glanced at my watch. It was now 6:00 a.m. We had been on scene almost six and a half hours. Harry and I were covered with dirt and oil. We both sank into a chair and stared at one another. "Son of a bitch," was all Harry had to say.

Nobody really expected Jim to survive. But he made it through the initial surgery, which lasted over ten hours. His ICU course was rocky and fraught with complications, and he nearly died many times, yet he had the tenacity to hang in there and was discharged five months later. Everyone was ecstatic.

A year later, Morgan Hill CDF called us. "We're going to have a party for Jim Henderson next week, and we'd really like you guys to come, especially the crew that was on that night."

As Harry and I walked in the door, there was a man supporting his right side with a cane. I didn't recognize him, but he walked directly up to Harry and shook his hand enthusiastically. Other than the limp, he looked perfectly healthy.

"I remember you," Jim said to Harry. "You were the guy that stuck that tube in my nose." They both laughed. "I want to thank you. You helped save my life. I owe you one." He turned to me. "And I remember you, too," he said simply. "I remember you holding me when I was trapped. I was afraid the truck was going to catch fire, but I figured as long as you were there with me, I was going to be OK. I can't tell you how alone I was, being stuck in there. I knew you would help me. Thank you." He hugged me tightly. Somebody snapped a picture at that moment.

I will always treasure it.

Into the Dead Zone

Rain poured off the eaves of CALSTAR quarters, where we had been comfortably watching the Sunday afternoon football game. Tim shook his head doubtfully as he hung up the phone to the weather service. "Well, I don't know if we can make it to Pacheco Pass, but we can go and try." Both Sarah and I groaned. We struggled into our rain gear and trudged out to the helicopter.

We affectionately refer to Pacheco Pass as Blood Alley. It's a two-lane, winding mountain road that connects the San Joaquin Valley to the south end of the Santa Clara Valley. The fifty-miles-per-hour speed limit is ignored by most vehicles, including hoards of monstrous semi trucks. The carnage has significantly decreased in the past several years with the place- ment of concrete barriers between the lanes of traffic, but there is still some pretty impressive trauma to be found there.

As we lifted off, Sarah rang up dispatch. "This is CALSTAR One. We are lifting at 13:32 hours en route to scene. Ready to copy information. Please advise CDF: Do not delay transport, as we're not sure weather will permit us to get to the scene." This was the usual drill when we flew in heavy clouds or fog. If the paramedics on the scene had the patient packaged, they would head to the hospital by ground rather than wasting precious time waiting for us. If we weren't able to get to the scene in time, we sometimes met the ambulance halfway.

"CALSTAR One, will advise CDF," dispatch replied. "You are going to Pacheco Pass, unknown exact location. No one is on scene yet. The reporting party is a passerby who is currently on cellphone with the CHP. Fire and medic are en route. You will be talking to Morgan Hill CDF on local net."

We settled into the flight, keeping quiet as Tim maneuvered through the rain. We were meeting our minimums— an altitude of eight hundred feet and one mile visibility—but if it got any worse, we would have to abort the flight. This could be frustrating, but we weren't going to do any good if we got in trouble and became an incident ourselves. I looked out at the threatening clouds and watched the altimeter discreetly—an extra pair of eyes always helps the pilot in rough weather.

We carefully threaded our way down the Santa Clara Valley, keeping CDF apprised of our progress. All we were told was the fire units and the medics were somewhere in the deep canyon of the pass, and we should be able to contact them as we approached. If we could see them below, that wouldn't be a problem, but for the most part, Pacheco Pass was a radio dead zone. Radio signals can only transmit in a straight line, which is difficult or impossible in remote places surrounded by mountains. To get around this problem, transmitters are usually built on the tops of tall buildings or on mountain peaks, so signals traveling upward can be retransmitted outward and downward. At the time of this incident, however, Pacheco Pass didn't have a transmitter, leaving us incommunicado.

To our surprise, we actually made it to the pass. Sarah began methodically making radio calls on the frequency the units were supposed to be using, but no one answered. She tried again, this time on the local frequency. Again, no luck. We discussed our options as Tim flew several large, lazy circles just below the pass, over Casa de Fruita, the last rest stop along the highway.

Finally, we agreed on a plan and Sarah keyed up the mike. "CDF, this is CALSTAR One. How do you copy?" There was no response. She tried again. "CDF, this is CALSTAR One transmitting in the blind. We are currently over Casa de Fruita and have no radio contact with the ground units. We will proceed up the canyon until we either find the incident or become unable to proceed due to weather. In that case, we will return to Casa de Fruita and land in the field abeam from the rest stop and await the ambulance. Do you copy?" Some brief static was the only reply. "Well, we might as well go take a look. We can't talk to anybody anyway."

"OK," said Tim. "Everybody with eyes out. We're outta here if this gets any worse." We all nodded and Tim turned the aircraft up toward the pass and followed the road, flying low and slow. The top of the pass was obscured by clouds, and none of us thought we'd get far. We searched the road for either the fire trucks or the ambulance, but saw no evidence of them. Sarah was broadcasting on the local frequency all along, but had no idea if anyone was hearing her.

About five miles up the canyon, we saw an overturned car in the ditch and a woman wildly gesturing to us. We were near a lookout point called Lover's Leap, and there was no fire truck or ambulance anywhere. "This is the damndest thing," Tim said. "Where could they be? We haven't passed them, and yet here's the accident." He looked back at us. "What do you think? We can land in the parking lot for Lover's Leap—there's plenty of room."

"Well, we're here, and we've got an LZ," I said. "Sarah, you'll have to stay with the helicopter for security until Tim can shut it down. Then bring all the packaging stuff and meet me over by the car. Tim, what do we do if the weather gets worse?"

"I'll hit the siren if it looks like we're about to get clouded in here, and we'll do the best we can. If we can't get out, at least you can have the patient in here getting care until the ambulance arrives or the weather lifts. I'll keep trying to raise dispatch or CDF, or anybody else."

After we landed, I stood outside the aircraft in the rain, pulling together as much of the packaging equipment as I could carry and tucking the portable radio into my jacket. I started for the four-lane highway, wondering how I was going to cross. We had attracted some attention from landing the helicopter, and the traffic had slowed down to take a look. I held up my hand, stopping traffic, and ran across the first two lanes. The opposite lanes were a different story—the cars and trucks were whizzing around a blind curve, oblivious to the rain. Then, when they saw the overturned vehicle, they would slam on their brakes, narrowly avoiding rear-ending the car in front. I waited for a break in the traffic, then made a treacherous run for it, crawling over the flimsy highway divider and nearly getting hit by a truck.

The woman was screaming as I headed down to the overturned car. "You have to get my babies! They're hurt and I can't get them out!" I got down on my knees and peered into the car. One little girl, who looked to be about four, was lying on what used to be the ceiling of the car, crying. A baby about six months old was still strapped in her infant seat, dangling upside down.

"What happened?" I asked, dumping all my gear on the ground.

"I came around this bend, and there was this car. I tried to swerve, but I lost control and rolled over. Oh, please, help my babies."

"Are you hurt?" I asked, looking at a cut on her forehead. "How did you get out?"

"I'm fine, I crawled out a window," she said.

I leaned down and peered into the car again. The four-year-old had a reassuring cry, but the baby was unnervingly quiet. I reached in and touched her. She had a pulse and was breathing, but didn't respond to my touch, an ominous sign. What was I supposed to do now? It was unusual for us to be the first and only EMS people on scene of an accident, and we had limited resources, but we would have to make do. Across the road, Tim was shutting down the engines on the helicopter, and Sarah was about to cross the highway, loaded down with backboards and collars. When she saw the patients were children, she sped up to a trot.

By now, several drivers had stopped to help. Two of them were off-duty police officers, and as Sarah got over the divider, one of them hiked up the road to stop the traffic.

I spoke to the four-year-old. "Sweetie, you're OK. I want you to just lie down, and we'll get you and your sister out soon." With the help of the other police officer and Sarah, we slid her gently onto the backboard and pulled her out of the car. "Now stay real still, OK?" We gently secured her onto the board and laid her on the roadway, now that the traffic had been stopped. Sarah then wiggled into the twisted car, and took a look at the baby, who was clearly the more injured of the two. Gently holding the child, we unlatched the seat belt and brought the whole car seat out with the little girl still strapped in.

"Should we leave her in the car seat?" Sarah asked. "At least she's secure there. We can strap it directly onto the litter."

"I'd like to, but I'm afraid we won't have good access to her airway. Maybe we can carry her to the helicopter in the seat and package her onto the litter when we get there. At any rate, we need to get her out of here—she's soaking wet, and this rain is getting worse."

Sarah agreed and left to load the four-year-old onto the helicopter. I did a quick assessment while Sarah was gone. The baby had a lump on her head and dark bruising around the right eye, which can indicate severe hemorrhaging. But her airway was unobstructed, she was breathing OK, and had reasonably good pulses. There was really nothing we could do except package her, start an IV, keep her warm and get her to Stanford, the closest available pediatric trauma center. I got her ready to cross the road.

"Where do I go?" the mother asked. "Can I come with you?"

Although all we could see was a cut forehead, this woman needed medical attention. It was quite possible she had hidden injuries she was masking (she did, after all, flip her car at highway speed), which made her a major trauma patient despite appearing fine. We only had two litters and the children needed them, but we couldn't leave this woman here in the rain with no transportation to Stanford, and we couldn't appropriately treat her on the helicopter. Then I flashed on a plan.

"Listen, I have an unusual idea." I explained to her the lack of space on the helicopter, and why we couldn't transport her as a patient. "If you're willing, what we'll do is sign you out against medical advice, then you can ride in the front seat with the pilot as a passenger rather than a patient. You can check yourself into ER when we get to Stanford."

This was highly unorthodox, and something a flight nurse

really shouldn't do. I was asking her to sign a piece of paper acknowledging that she was declining care, releasing us from liability. If she ended up having a serious injury, she could probably have taken us to court to argue that she wasn't in a rational frame of mind. But alone on the scene in the driving rain, with two pediatric patients, I decided to play the odds.

"Of course I'll do that," she said. "Really, I'm fine." We started across the roadway, carefully carrying the baby in the car seat. Sarah was watching me quizzically, not sure why the mother was with me. I explained my plan and checked with Tim to make sure we could do it with weight and balance. He did some quick calculations and assured us it would work. Then, as we were moving the baby onto the litter, an ambulance pulled up.

"Where the hell have you guys been?" we asked the medics as they ran over.

"You're not going to believe this, but there is another accident just up the road, which is where everybody is. There's already one ambulance there—we're the second unit to respond. They're worried about you 'cause you never made it. Last they heard was you were at Casa de Fruita, and when the CHP looked for you there, you were gone. Everybody's looking for you. And what's all this?"

We filled them in and they agreed to our scheme—they needed to get up to the other accident and didn't have time to take the mother to Stanford. We were still in the radio dead zone, so we couldn't let anybody know the strange turn of events, nor could this ambulance. We quickly loaded everybody into the aircraft and, after strapping mom in the front seat, got airborne.

The baby was in worse shape then we had thought. She was quite shocky and needed fluids quickly. We started lines and hooked her up to the monitors, trying to keep calm, since her mom could hear everything we said on the intercom. My anxiety grew as we worked on the baby.

Suddenly the beeper on my belt began to vibrate. I quickly looked down, and saw the pager code we never wanted to see: 911. This was a company-wide page that indicated that one of our three aircraft had gone down. As in *crashed*.

My heart dropped in my shoes. I knew CALSTAR Two was off on an interfacility flight, so it could only have been them. "Oh my God, you guys. Harry and J.B. are in trouble. I just got a 911 page." Everyone grew very somber, very quiet.

Tim was the first to speak. "We can't do anything about that right now. We have to get out of this pass, and you guys have a sick little kid to deal with. Let's keep ourselves in the ball game till we can get out of this, OK?" Sarah and I looked at one another and returned to our small patient.

As we emerged from the pass, Sarah was able to finally reach CDF Morgan Hill. "CDF, this is CALSTAR One. We are unable to contact our dispatch. We are currently en route to Stanford with two pediatric patients on board. Could you please notify Stanford of our ETA? And could you please contact our dispatch and let them know of our route?"

"CALSTAR One, this is CDF. Are we glad to hear from you. We will certainly advise both your dispatch and Stanford. Give us a call when you get there." None of us had connected the dots yet; we were entirely too busy with our patients.

After we landed at Stanford I called dispatch, dreading what I was about to hear. As I was waiting to be connected, one of the unit clerks came into the room. "Hey, CALSTAR, you have a call on line two. She seems pretty upset."

We all looked at each other, and I slowly picked up the phone. It was Beth, the administrator on call. "Where in the hell have you guys been?" she demanded. "I almost had a heart attack. We thought you had crashed on Pacheco Pass. I have the whole company, including the board and the president, headed for the office right now. What happened to you guys?" She seemed close to tears.

I still hadn't quite gotten the picture. "Are J.B. and Harry OK?" I asked. "Where are they? Were they hurt? How bad was it?"

"What are you talking about?"

It took almost a day to sort out what had happened. Two fire engines, a CHP patrol car, and an ambulance had entered Pacheco Pass and lost all radio contact with their bases. They activated CALSTAR, as there were reports of major injuries. As we approached the pass, CDF was able to hear our last transmission: that we would proceed up the pass, and if weather became bad, we would turn around and meet the ambulance at Casa de Fruita. We were unaware that the message had reached them.

When we stumbled upon the overturned car, we assumed this was what we had been dispatched for. But it turns out that the first crash was several miles away and no one knew about this mother and her children, which explains why the fire department and paramedics were nowhere in sight.

In the meantime, having heard our radio transmission and figuring the weather would force us to turn around quickly, the CHP sent a second patrol car to Casa de Fruita to land the helicopter. When we didn't show up there, it notified all the dispatch centers that no one had seen or heard from us in more than 30 minutes of bad weather. That's when CALSTAR set in motion the downed-aircraft policy.

When the dust finally settled, both children pulled through and they installed a radio transmitter above Pacheco Pass, something that should have been done years ago. During my ten years in the air, I never got another 911 page.

Hard Lessons

BETH and I were taking our usual afternoon siesta at Camp CALSTAR, enjoying the warm summer sun. We had been on a scene call earlier in the day and the patient's injuries were relatively minor. But I had that flying feeling, and the sense that something evil was looming.

Simultaneously the beepers went off and the phone rang. I swung off the bed, grabbing the receiver. "CALSTAR One, you've been dispatched for a motor vehicle accident on Pacheco Pass. The map coordinates are Santa Clara County page 64, grid B4. You will be talking to Morgan Hill CDF on local net, who will direct you to the frequency the accident is working. Be advised this is a multi-casualty incident."

"Copy that. Our ETA is seventeen minutes after liftoff," I said, struggling into my flight suit.

As we flew toward the scene, Beth, who was flying second-ary, started making radio calls to contact the ground units. "CDF Morgan Hill, this is CALSTAR One. Ready to copy fre-quency for ground contact on Pacheco Pass incident."

"CALSTAR One, this is Morgan Hill CDF. Your ground contact will be Engine 4145 on this frequency. How do you copy?"

"That's a good copy for CALSTAR One, thanks." We were still five minutes away, and although we could hear the radio traffic from the scene, we couldn't talk to them until we were past the last ridge line, when we'd be essentially on top of the accident. That wouldn't give us much time. It really didn't matter. We'd know the story soon enough.

As we were flying up the last valley toward the pass, we could see the traffic backing up below. "This one must be pretty bad," Beth said. "They're not letting anybody through." We kept following the road, and as we came around a corner, the accident popped into view. There were two cars on the side of the road completely trashed, and another one rolled in a ditch. A double-trailer semi truck was jackknifed across the road, completely blocking traffic.

I had to giggle a bit. "I'll bet CHP is going nuts." The Cali-fornia Highway Patrol seems to have only one goal — to keep traffic moving at all costs. This accident must be giving them ulcers, I thought, as it was obvious this road would be blocked up a good while.

Beth grinned and keyed up the mike. "Engine 4145, this is CALSTAR One. We are overhead incident. Where would you like us?"

On a scene call, establishing an LZ was usually the respon-sibility of the fire department. They would radio to tell us exactly where on the scene they wanted us, point out any obstructions like power lines, poles or light standards, advise us of wind direction and speed, and indicate the type of surface we'd be landing on. This time a familiar voice answered us. "Uh, CALSTARrrrrssss, this is Engine 4145. I'm right here. Come on down."

"Oh God," Beth muttered. "It's Frank."

Frank was a firefighter with the California Division of Forestry (CDF), a well-trained group whose main duty is to battle summer wildfires in isolated areas, as well as manage areas that are too sparsely populated to maintain a municipal firehouse. The core staff is a remarkably talented group, and in the summer it's supplemented by young people who are paid only a paltry wage for the grueling and dangerous work of fighting wildfires. They do this to gain experience in hopes of landing a job as a municipal firefighter—or possibly from some twisted sense of responsibility to the environment. In the off-season, these departments run a skeleton staff of full-timers and respond to county calls that are out of the jurisdiction of neighboring fire departments. On the whole, these men and women are heroes, risking their lives for very little compensation.

But Frank was different. He was one of the good ol' boys the department didn't have the heart to retire. Certainly he was a decent and delightful man, but utterly incapable of setting up a landing zone. Our first clue to Frank's incompetence was his insistence upon referring to us as "CALSTARrrrrssss."

Beth attempted to decode what Frank meant by being "right here." More than twenty yellow fire coats milled about below us. "Engine 4145, this is CALSTAR. We see quite a few firefighters on scene, and we're not sure which one is you."

"CALSTARrrrrssss, I'm not at the accident. I'm in the green field down the road." We looked around at green fields stretching for miles in all directions.

Beth tried again. "Engine 4145, are you north or south of the scene, and do you have any landmarks nearby? We do not have a visual on you."

"CALSTARrrrrssss, I'm in a green field with a white fence. You're on my left," he replied.

Well, that certainly helped. All the fields were green with white fences, and which way was his left? "Engine 4145, do you have us in sight? If so, please tell us to turn right or left. I repeat, we do not have a visual on you."

This time there was a slight pause. "Nope. Can't see you. But I can hear you, I think."

Tim, our pilot, was getting exasperated. "Beth, let me try. Maybe I can get this guy to understand." He keyed up the mike. "Engine 4145. This is the CALSTAR pilot. We are currently circling the scene. We have green fields with white fences stretching for miles in both directions. I am going to head south on Highway 152, away from the accident, towards Hollister. Are we headed for you?"

"Yup," was Frank's only reply.

"OK, everybody," Tim said, keying up the intercom. "Look for a dipshit in a field holding a radio. That's got to be him." We flew on in silence for a few minutes, with all eyes straining to pick up a fire engine off the road.

"Dipshit in field at two o'clock," Beth said. "I got him on the right side. Sure enough, he's in a green field with a white fence."

"Well, I'm glad he got something right," Tim said. He swung the helicopter to the right to take a look. "All right, I have him. I'm going to try and get landing zone instructions." He keyed the radio to the ground. "Engine 4145, we believe we are overhead your location. Do you have us in sight?"

"CALSTARrrrrssss, I can see you now. Yup, this is your LZ.

Come on down." I could see him waving his arms and point-ing to the small field where he was standing.

"Engine 4145, do you have any obstructions and can you give us an idea of wind direction and speed?"

"I don't think there's any wires, and there sure is a pretty strong breeze down here," our nemesis replied.

"Tim, there's a flag over there," Beth said, pointing to a nearby barn. That would give us an idea of what the winds were doing. None of us believed Frank when he said there were no obstructions.

"Yeah, I just saw that," Tim said. "I've been in here before, so I feel pretty comfortable. Let's make a quick pass to take a look. But everybody keep heads up on final, OK?"

As we circled, all looked clear. Tim turned final and keyed up the mike. "Engine 4145, we are on short final. Please clear the LZ."

Frank continued to stand in the middle of the LZ, wildly gesturing at his feet, exactly where we needed to land.

"4145, you are standing where the helicopter needs to be. Please move off the LZ."

"Oh, yeah. OK." Frank ambled off toward his fire truck.

As we landed, I grabbed the adult trauma bag. "You don't think we're getting a pediatric patient, do you?" I asked Beth. Our pediatric supplies were in a separate bag in the back.

"No," she said. "We've drilled it into all the fire depart-ments to give us a heads-up with pedi patients. Even Frank knows that." I nodded, unbelted, and climbed down the skid to the ground. I walked over to where Frank was standing.

"Hi, Frank," I said. "How are you doing?" I was tempted to give him a lecture on how to land a helicopter, but stopped myself. This wasn't the place.

"Good to see ya again," he replied. "Hey, are you guys coming to the barbecue next week?" he asked, clearly unconcerned with our approaching patient.

An ambulance came around the corner, with lights and siren on, and pulled heavily into the field. I glanced over at the helicopter, which was still running. Beth had the litter out and was standing and talking with Tim. I motioned to her and she nodded. I walked to the back of the ambulance, opened the door, then stood dumbly staring at the interior.

Mother of God, it was a toddler. In full arrest. I looked down at my adult trauma bag, which was now completely useless. Frank stood beside me, grinning.

I carefully turned to him, trying to control my rage. I enunciated through gritted teeth. "Go to my partner, NOW, and tell her to COME IMMEDIATELY. With the PEDIATRIC BAG. Do you understand?" Frank nodded vigorously and scurried off as I climbed into the back of the ambulance.

It was a little girl, probably about three. One medic was assisting her ventilations, and the other was doing chest compressions. I did a quick initial assessment. Both legs were splayed out at unnatural angles, with bones viciously sticking out of the skin. She was just lying on the gurney, with no packaging done. Her face was covered with blood, and her skin had a bluish tinge. On the opposite bench her mother was screaming.

I squeezed past the paramedic doing compressions to the head. "Do you want me to take over ventilations?" I asked.

"Yeah," he said. "Sorry about this. This is a passenger who was hit head-on by a semi truck at around sixty miles per hour. She was in the back seat with no belt, and when the car rolled, she was ejected. We didn't even realize she was there until the mother here woke up and started yelling for her. We found her about 150 feet from the car in a ditch. Initially, she had a faint pulse and gasping respirations, but those are gone now. We see injuries to the head, chest, abdomen, and the obvious extremity stuff. We used up all of our equipment with the other patients, and then the incident commander just dumped her on us."

Beth appeared at the ambulance door and surveyed the scene before her. She didn't miss a beat. She crawled in, handing the pedi bag up to me, and I quickly gave her the story. "We need to intubate her now," I said. "You guys start packaging her while I get my stuff together."

"Do you guys have a backboard?" Beth asked the medic.

"No, I was just explaining to your partner," he replied, continuing CPR. "Nobody knew she was there until all of the equipment was used up on the other patients at the scene." Beth looked around the ambulance, then grabbed a short board that is used to provide a firm surface for adult CPR. It would be just long enough to support the little body. She looked up at me. "Are you ready to tube now, or can we roll her onto the board first?"

"Let's get her on the board first so you guys can finish packaging her while I do the tube," I answered. "Is everybody ready? On three." We gently logrolled her onto the board, holding the cervical spine aligned, and with Beth trying in vain to support the horribly disfigured legs. The mother had stopped screaming and was intently watching. I grabbed the laryngoscope and gently placed it into the child's mouth, which was filled with blood. "I need suction," I said, and held up my hand, hoping the medic or Beth would anticipate the need and be able to help while I kept my eyes on the girl. There was no suction. I looked up and saw the medic frantically pounding on the switch, but it was not responding.

"It's not working," he said. "I can't believe this."

I resumed bagging with the mask. "Beth, I can't get this tube without suction to clear out all this blood. I'm just going to hand-ventilate her until we get to the aircraft. We'll do it en route. That OK with you?" We both knew this child had no chance for survival, but we couldn't give up on her, especially with the mother in the ambulance witnessing this awful spectacle.

"Sounds like that's our only option," she said. "I'll do compressions until we get en route."

We started off to the aircraft, which was still running. Only ten minutes had elapsed since we had landed, but it seemed like an eternity. As we loaded the girl in, I yelled at Tim. "As soon as we get airborne, call dispatch and tell them we're coming with a three-year-old blunt traumatic arrest. We're going to be too busy to give a report." He nodded his head and reached over to help load the litter.

In the air I started suctioning out her mouth and grabbed the laryngoscope, saying a brief prayer to the intubation gods. Thankfully, I could now see the vocal cords and was able to pass the endotracheal tube. As we started bagging her, her chest rose and fell with each breath, and our $ETCO_2$ detector turned a reassuring yellow, indicating the tube was in the right spot.

Beth, who had been doing compressions, reached over and switched us to hot mike, so we could talk over the intercom with hands free. "Do you want me to start an intraosseous line now?" An intraosseous line works like an IV, except that it's placed directly into the bone of young children. Young children's bone marrow is soft and vascular, so any fluids or medications are easily absorbed. And the bones are a much larger target than a tiny scalp or hand vein.

"Yeah," I nodded. "Looks like the only place to go is the right femur. Everything else is pulverized. I'll do compressions." She nodded. After the line was established, she gave the first round of medications and started pushing fluids. We checked the monitor. Where only a flat line had been, we now had a rhythm. "Do we have pulses?" I asked.

Beth reached down and felt for the femoral. "I don't believe it," she said. "We've got a pulse. Let me check a pressure. Stop compressions." To our amazement, it read 80/30. We were landing at the trauma center.

As we unloaded, the trauma team met us at the helipad. The trauma surgeon and pediatrician took a quick look at our patient. "We heard this was a blunt traumatic arrest," yelled the pediatrician over the noise of the rotor blades. "Did you get anything back en route?"

"It's hard to believe," I yelled back, "but we have a rhythm and a blood pressure." We ran into the trauma room, where the entire team swung into action. As they were hooking her up to the monitors, she arrested again. This time they did not get her back.

Later that day, we received a call from a CHP officer who was working the scene. His investigation was now being treated as a homicide. Apparently, mom had gotten into a fight with the boyfriend and, after drinking a pint of vodka, decided it was time to leave. She had "forgotten" to put the seat belt on her little girl.

Looking back, I know that even if we had landed routinely and hadn't needed to return to the helicopter for the pediatric bag, no intervention would have saved that girl. But we did learn an important lesson that day with Frank: *Never assume anything*. Since I didn't get the message on that flight, I learned it all over again some time later.

That particular night, the phone had jarred us awake at 3:00 a.m. Lunging for it, I managed to send both the phone and the bedside lamp crashing to the floor. "Where are we going?" I mumbled. Nancy was stumbling around the room in the dark, groping for her flight suit.

Elise, our dispatcher, informed us we were going to Yosemite General, a small hospital in the mountains near Yosemite National Park, more than an hour away. We were to pick up a patient and bring him back to Children's Hospital in Oakland. "You've been activated for a two-week-old infant with a diagnosis of oomphalitis," she said.

"Oomphalitis?" I asked. "What in heaven's name is that?"

"O-O-M-P-H-A-L-I-T-I-S," she spelled. "Apparently it's an infected bellybutton."

As I dressed, I mentally sorted through all the potentially disastrous or life-threatening pediatric conditions I could think of. Let's see—meningitis, congenital anomalies, trauma, respiratory infection, and shock. None of these possibly lethal conditions fit with an infected bellybutton. Sighing, I reached for my flight suit and jump boots. I didn't see any way we could turf this call, as the sky was clear and starlit—perfect flying weather. Occasionally, Children's Hospital would call us to transport non-critical patients, and in keeping with CAL-STAR's philosophy of "you call, we haul," we were obliged even when it seemed an unnecessary use of an emergency resource.

We headed out to the helicopter muttering obscenities. "What are we going after?" Nancy asked, wiping the sleep out of her eyes.

"You'll never believe this," I said. "It's a two-week-old with an infected bellybutton."

Nancy was one of the newer flight nurses, born and raised in New York. She spoke with a heavy Long Island accent and had an attitude to match. "You gotta be kidding me," she said.

"These guys dragged me out of bed for a goddamn infected bellybutton? What is this shit?" J.B. wasn't happy about piloting a long middle-of-the-night flight either.

The three of us climbed into the helicopter and lifted off. The flight was quiet, punctuated only by the necessary communications. We flew over the San Joaquin Valley, then up into the foothills of the Sierra, where Tuolumne is located. I was still puzzled by the bellybutton and wondered if maybe I was missing something here. I pulled out the pediatric transport resource book to see if oomphalitis was discussed. It wasn't, which meant that when we got back to Children's some first-year resident was going to get an earful from me regarding the appropriate use of an emergency helicopter.

An hour later, we landed at the local airport, because Yosemite General Hospital doesn't have a helipad. We had called an ambulance for the twenty-minute drive, and the crew that met us looked like they had been through a meat grinder. Their uniforms were wrinkled and smelly, and they regarded us with bloodshot eyes.

"What are you here for?" one of them asked wearily as we loaded all our equipment onto their litter.

"An infected bellybutton," I replied. Disgust clouded his face.

"Let me get this right," he said. "You got us out of bed at this ungodly hour for an infected bellybutton?"

"I'm sorry," I said. "This call will definitely be flagged for review with the Children's transport committee." The only reply was a grunt from the front of the ambulance.

When we arrived at Yosemite General, we were met at the back door by a very nervous young pediatrician. He slung his arm around my shoulder, propelling me toward an exam room. He pushed the chart into my hands, speaking rapidly.

"For now, all of his labs are normal, but I'm considering repeating the blood gases to see if there is a change. I've started him on triple antibiotics, but we may send you with another dose. I'm really worried about this kid. Do you think you can expedite this transport?"

"Why don't you let us take a look at him first," I suggested. Patience is not one of my virtues, especially at 3:00 a.m., and I was already exasperated with this nervous little man. I looked over at Nancy, who just rolled her eyes.

As I walked into the exam room, all of my expectations were confirmed. There, in his mother's arms, was the cutest, pinkest little baby I had ever seen, sucking contentedly on a pacifier. He turned toward us as we entered the room, then concentrated again on his Nuk. His parents, obviously worried, watched us carefully.

"Is he going to be OK?" the young mother asked. I could see the panic in her eyes, which was clearly being made worse by the anxious pediatrician hovering behind me.

"From where I stand, he looks wonderful," I replied. "Could you put him down on the gurney so we can get a good look at him, please?" She laid the baby down and I carefully unwrapped him. His skin signs were great, his pulses were bounding, and his vital signs were all completely normal, including his temperature. So far as I could see, this little guy was in better shape than I was. When I took off his diaper, I saw what all the fuss was about. Surrounding the umbilicus was a pocket of pus, and the stump itself was red, with a small amount of greenish drainage. The rest of the child, however, was in splendid form. His IV was in place and infusing well, and he had received the necessary antibiotics.

I turned to the parents, who were watching us intently. "He's going to be fine," I said. "We'll just run him down to

Children's, and they'll take very good care of him. He looks like a special little boy. Your first, right?"

They nodded. "He was kind of unexpected," the dad said. "But you know, you get pretty attached to these guys."

We got busy hooking the baby to all the monitors. While Nancy finished packaging the little boy, I called Children's to give them a report. To add to my frustration, nobody could find the night resident. I listened to annoying Muzak for ten minutes, impatiently tapping a pencil on the desk. Finally I hung up and called the ICU again. I spoke with the charge nurse and gave her a brief report of what we had seen. I told her to let the resident know we were en route, and if he had any further orders to contact us via dispatch.

When I got back to the exam room, Nancy had the baby all ready to go. We didn't take families on flights unless it was an unusual situation. There's not much room in the helicopter— they would have had to fly in the front seat, where they would have access to the flight controls, so the pilots considered it a safety issue. On the medical side, we didn't want the family there in case something went wrong. If the patient arrested, the family would be stuck in the helicopter with us, listening to everything we were doing, some of which can be pretty unnerving. And we'd need to concentrate on the patient without being distracted by a hysterical family member. One of the few times I did allow a parent to fly along, I ended up taking care of her as well. She became so violently airsick that we had to start an IV and give her medication to treat the nausea.

I reassured the parents and encouraged them to be careful on the treacherous drive out of the mountains. It would take them three or four hours to drive to Oakland. "As a matter of fact, why don't you go home and take a shower and pack a few things," I suggested. "The staff at the hospital can manage till you get there."

Our anxious pediatrician hovered in the background, occasionally imploring us to hurry, which only annoyed me further. We had only been there for twenty minutes, and we were moving as fast as we could. We certainly weren't going to dawdle. Our beds were waiting.

The grumpy ambulance crew took us back to the helicopter. The baby promptly fell asleep after liftoff. He woke up once and became a little fussy, but was quickly soothed with his pacifier. I found myself nodding off at one point, and shook my head to concentrate on our little patient.

When we arrived at Children's, I was a bit testy in giving my report to the staff. "I'm not sure why this guy had to come down by helicopter tonight, but here he is. His vital signs are stable, and his perfusion is great. We're going home. We'll call later and see how he's doing, OK?" I figured that by the time I made the call the baby would be out of the ICU.

As we were walking out of the ER, the early morning sun was just peeking through the Oakland Hills. "You know," Nancy said, "there's something depressing about watching a sunrise without an all-night party and an imminently righteous hangover to show for it."

"Or at least a righteous flight," I said.

J.B. was waiting for us at the helicopter.

"How's the baby doing?" he asked

"I'd say better than us," I replied. "Can we go home now?"

A day later I was back at CALSTAR still fuming at what seemed to me a wasteful flight. I was preparing to phone the transport coordinator at Children's and give her this opinion, but before doing that I wanted to call and see if the baby was already out on the floor, or perhaps even discharged as I expected. Dolores, the unit secretary answered the phone.

"Hi, Dolores. It's Janice from CALSTAR. How's things over there this morning?"

"It's really busy right now," she answered. "We've got dueling codes going on and everybody is going berserk." In medical jargon, a code—or code blue—is a cardiac arrest, and it also refers to the sequence of events we follow in trying to resuscitate the patient.

"Sorry to hear that. I'll make this short. Do you know where the baby is we brought down early yesterday morning? He had an infected bellybutton. From Yosemite."

"I hate to tell you this, but he's one of the codes. He arrested about twenty minutes ago."

The floor opened up and swallowed me. "Oh my God, Dolores, what happened?" I whispered.

"I don't know exactly. I think I heard somebody talking about florid septic shock. Does that make sense?"

I thanked her and hung up, realizing she was too busy to be chatting on the phone. Nancy, who was back with me for another shift, saw the expression on my face. "What happened?" she demanded.

"They're coding him. He's in septic shock." At that moment, I couldn't get any more words out. We had been bitching for the entire flight about this infected bellybutton. And now he was dying. Worse than that, I had reassured the parents that all was well, fine, no problem. Now they were sitting outside in the lounge waiting to hear if their firstborn son was dead.

In the end, our worst fears came true. The little boy died later that afternoon, despite aggressive, heroic efforts. It seems that an infected bellybutton in a newborn is a superhighway for bacteria to get into the central circulation. A very young child's immune system can't manage an onslaught of virulent bugs. The presence of such a large pocket of pus was an indication of how extensive his infection had gotten. The anxious pediatrician at Yosemite General had every reason for his concern.

I don't think we could or would have done anything differently from a medical standpoint—he got to a specialized pediatric hospital quickly. But this flight taught me another lesson: Never, ever cop an attitude. It only reveals your ignorance.

Blown Away on Interstate 5, and Other Stupid Human Tricks

Even after ten years in the air, and many more in hospital settings, I'm still surprised by the predicaments people can get themselves into when distracted by sex, alcohol or drugs.

My personal favorite came one winter evening when the thermometer had dropped to twenty-nine degrees. I snuggled deeper into my deliciously warm bed at CALSTAR quarters. Peering out the window, I saw a light film of frost covering the ground and trees, which shimmered in the moonlit night. In the bed next to me, Carrie slept soundly. Tim was in the next room, and the wall between us vibrated from his deep snoring.

The beeper gods would not allow such tranquility to last. Just as I was falling into a contented sleep, my pager went off. Swearing colorfully, I began dressing as I dialed dispatch. Kirstie picked it up on the first ring.

"Where are we going?" I asked.

"Sorry to get you out there tonight," she said. "You're headed out to San Joaquin County on Interstate 5. Two big rigs hit head-on, and they're calling it a multi-casualty incident. It's going to be on I-5 between Patterson and Crow's Landing. I'll get specific map coordinates and ground frequencies when you get en route, OK?"

"No problem. Give them a rough ETA of twenty minutes after we lift off, and check availability of Modesto Memorial North, if you would be so kind." I pulled on my flight suit over my bulky long underwear and grappled with the zipper. Tim was already in the helicopter cranking up, and Carrie and I headed out the door to join him.

The flight was quiet, punctuated only by the necessary radio communications. We flew through the saddle of Mount Diablo, through the Altamont Pass and then headed south over Interstate 5. The accident was supposed to be at least ten miles to the south. Finding it was a piece of cake—in the flat valley the beacons of the fire trucks were visible as soon as we got over the highway.

Carrie keyed up the radio, calling the IC, or incident commander. "I-5 IC, this is CALSTAR One. We have the scene in sight. Please give us landing zone instructions when we are overhead. Our ETA is three to four minutes."

"CALSTAR One, I-5 IC. All helicopter traffic will be on fire white, call sign Engine 1492. Copy your ETA. You will be transporting the driver of one of the semi trucks. He is still being extricated."

"CALSTAR One, switching to fire white now." She reached over and adjusted the radio to the new frequency, shaking her head. Switching the helicopter traffic to another frequency usually indicated a chaotic scene—there were so many units responding that one frequency couldn't handle all the radio traffic.

We circled the scene twice to get a general idea of the incident. The accident was impressive, and a good lesson in basic physics. Two thirty-ton juggernauts of steel hitting head on at seventy miles per hour can produce some rather impressive damage. The two trucks lay on their sides, as if they were colossal dinosaurs contracted in a death grip. Twisted hunks of metal debris were spread over a half-mile. Both cabs were unrecognizable from the impact and it seemed extraordinary that anyone could survive such carnage. We could see streams of sparks flying into the air as the firefighters sawed through the metal to release our patient from inside his cab. From the air, the scene had the surreal quality of an elaborate movie set.

We landed on a grassy median north of the accident and found the incident commander shouting instructions into his portable radio. Between the roar of the helicopter jet engines and the screeching din of the Jaws of Life, it was difficult to hear anything. "Which one do you want us to take?" I yelled, wondering what kind of mangled remains we might be presented with.

"The one over there," he shouted, pointing to the cab that was lying in the middle of the road. Carrie and I carefully picked our way through the field of metal chunks of truck toward the paramedics who were pulling our patient out of the twisted wreck onto a backboard.

"Hi, I'm Janice from CALSTAR," I yelled into the paramedic's ear. "What's the story?" He screamed the report back into my ear while the medics continued strapping the patient onto the backboard and placing an oxygen mask on him, and I started pulling our IV and intubation equipment from the trauma bag.

"This guy was the driver of this truck," he said, gesturing to one of the mangled cabs. "He's got a head injury, bruising over his chest, and abdominal abrasions. He doesn't recall the incident and has repetitive speech. I can't hear breath sounds 'cause of all the noise. He also has some extremity trauma—his left wrist and left leg were angulated. We have those splinted. Sorry, we didn't have access to start an IV."

I leaned over the patient and started a primary survey, noting he wore only a torn shirt. I assumed the medics had cut off his pants to evaluate his lower extremities, a common practice. "What's your name?" I asked.

"Bob," he replied. This was good—it meant his airway was intact enough to speak, and his brain must be getting enough of a blood pressure. His radial pulse was rapid and thready, but if I could feel it that meant his systolic BP was at least eighty.

"Where do you hurt?" I asked next, palpating his chest, abdomen and pelvis.

"Bob, Bob, Bob," was his reply.

Well, OK, at least he was talking. I did a quick secondary survey, which revealed, in addition to the broken limbs, chest injuries that would threaten his breathing, a rigid abdomen, which suggested internal bleeding, and a sickening crunch as I gently rocked his pelvis. This man needed to be in the capable hands of a hospital trauma team quickly. It was too noisy to try to listen to his breath sounds, so I wrapped a tourniquet around his good arm in anticipation of starting an IV in the helicopter, and prepared to get the patient loaded.

"Bob," I yelled, "you've been in an accident, and we're going to take you to the hospital so they can get you all fixed up, OK?"

"Bob, Bob, Bob, Bob."

I shook my head and handed him over to Carrie. As I headed off to the helicopter, the incident commander grabbed my shoulder. "Where are you taking him? His wife was in the cab, too, but doesn't seem to be hurt too badly. We're taking her to Tracy Community Hospital to get checked out. She wants to get to wherever you're going as soon as possible."

"We're going to Modesto Memorial North," I yelled, and then headed to the helicopter to prepare for our patient's arrival.

As Carrie loaded Bob into the aircraft, I quickly got him set up on all the monitors. His blood pressure was low, and his heart rate was 150. Thankfully, his blood-oxygen saturations were in the high nineties, indicating his oxygenation hadn't yet been compromised by his chest injuries. Through it all, our patient continued his mantra: "Bob, Bob, Bob, Bob."

I didn't want to wipe out his airway reflexes by intubating him now. That would have to be done eventually, but to do it in the field with a patient who is still marginally awake requires a rapid sequence induction, or RSI. We give the patient a sedative and then a medication that paralyzes him, allowing us to overcome coughing and gagging when we stuff the breathing tube into his trachea. This would take away his ability to breathe on his own. Moreover, the hospital trauma team would need to do a neurological evaluation, which isn't possible if the patient is intubated, sedated and paralyzed. Finally, our friend Bob had a bull neck, a receding jaw, and probably a stomach full of Big Macs, making intubation difficult and aspiration—breathing in his own vomit—a likelihood. In any case, his oxygen saturations were in good shape, so I didn't want to start looking for trouble.

Our flight to the trauma center was quite busy, as we started Bob's IVs and began pushing fluids into him. As soon as Carrie got the IV established, I switched the radio to the receiving hospital and gave a brief report.

"Modesto Memorial, CALSTAR One. We are currently en route to your facility with an ETA of twelve minutes. On board we have an approximately forty-five-year-old patient who was the belted driver of a semi that was hit head-on by another semi truck, both traveling at sixty to seventy miles per hour. Our patient required an approximately twenty-minute extrication. We are seeing a head injury with repetitive speech, a small flail segment on the left chest, and a rigid abdomen. His pelvis is unstable, and there is no priapism." Priapism—that is, an abnormally persistent erection—can indicate a spinal injury, so Bob's flaccid state was a good thing. I explained Bob's other injuries and his vital signs, and got the OK from Modesto Memorial.

When we landed at the helipad, several members of the trauma team were there to meet us and we offloaded the patient with the helicopter still running. He continued chanting "Bob, Bob, Bob, Bob" as we rushed him to where the rest of the team waited. I gave a report as they launched into their choreographed routine.

As we pulled out our litter and supplies, I found the trauma coordinator standing by the door, watching the resuscitation. It was my old friend Diana, whom I had worked with at Seton Hospital's ER.

"Hi, Diana. How's things in the Modesto trauma business?"

Bob was now screaming in the background, adding to the cacophony of the trauma room. "BOB, BOB, BOB, BOB," he yelled as the nurse drew blood and the physician rocked his pelvis.

"Busy as usual," she said. "How is this guy?"

"Pretty sick, I'd say. Quite verbal though. Hey, listen, the incident commander on scene told me they found his wife with him in the cab and, miraculously, she isn't hurt badly. They're taking her to Tracy Community to get her checked out, but she'll probably be here later tonight. You'll take care of it, won't you?"

"Of course. Call me in the morning and I'll let you know how it all goes."

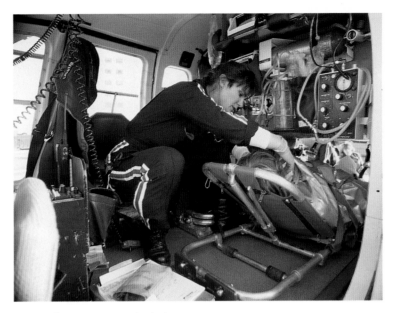

Caring for a patient in the helicopter.

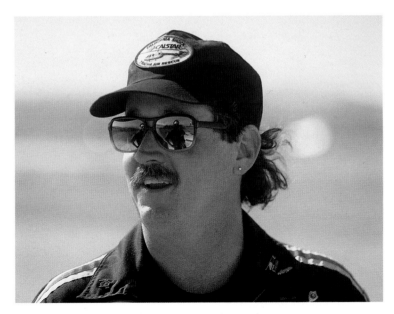

Harry—one of the best flight nurses in the profession.

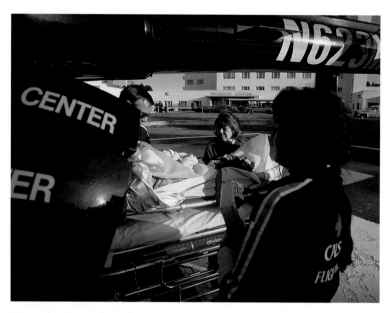

Harry (my Danny) evaluating a trauma patient.

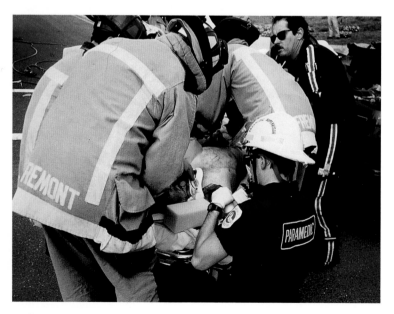

Unloading a patient.

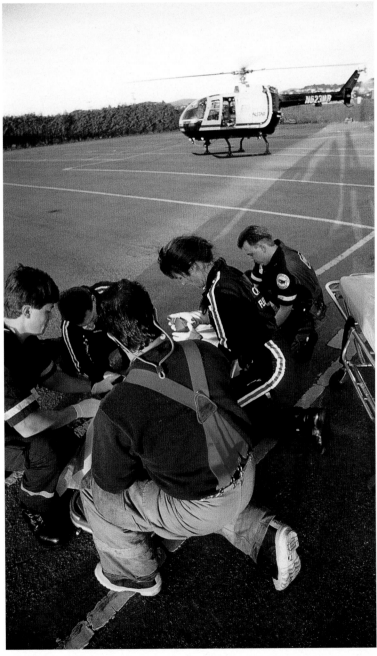

Above: Packaging a patient prior to loading into the helicopter.
Following page: The whole team (CALSTAR group photo).

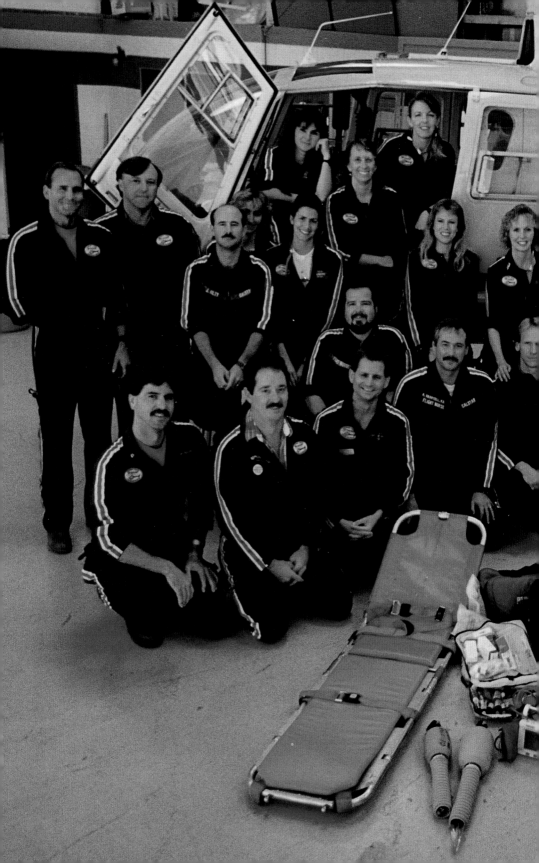

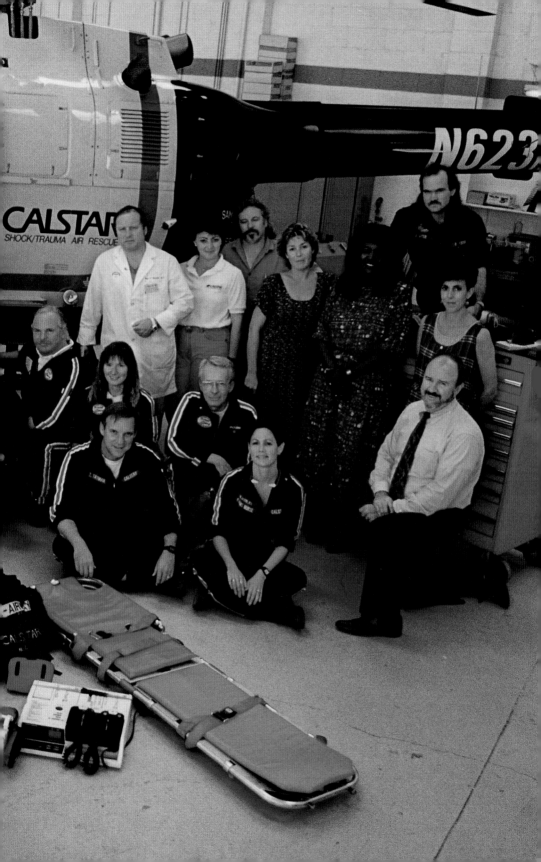

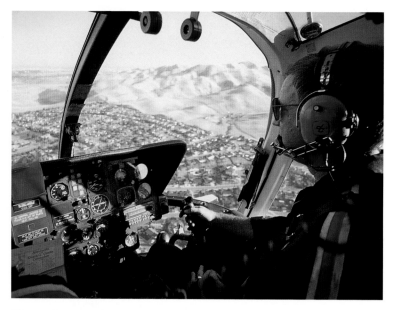

Tim at the controls.

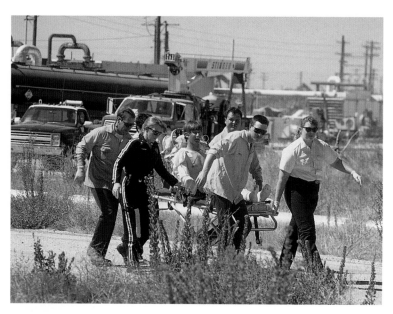

Linda loading a patient.

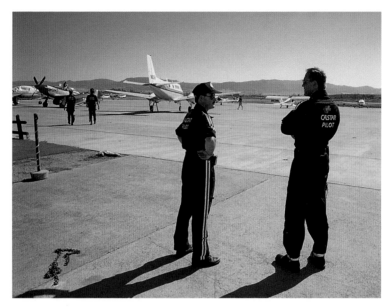

JB and Dave at the airport.

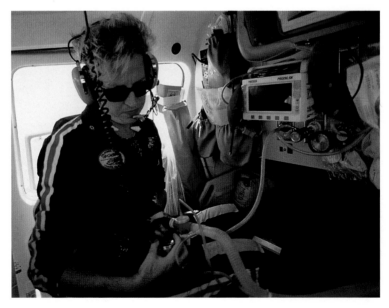

My Rosie.

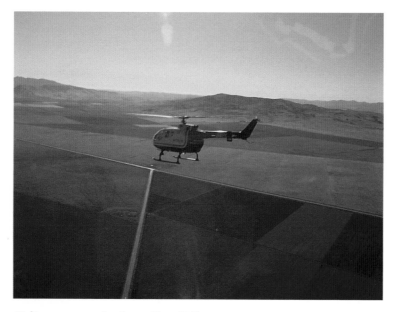

Helicopter over the Santa Clara Valley.

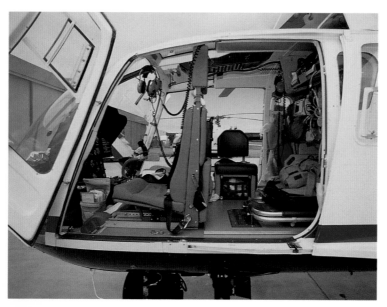

Interior of helicopter.

The next morning, Diana called me before I had a chance to track her down. "Janice, you aren't going to believe this one."

"Is Bob doing OK?" I asked.

"Well, he was a mess, and he was in the OR until 5:00 a.m. He's going to do fine. But there's more."

"Oh?"

"Remember you told me his wife was with him?"

"Yes. Did she get there OK?"

"Oh, she sure did. She showed up around 3:00 a.m., a little bruised, but doing fine. She was very concerned about Bob and insisted on staying awake all night waiting for him. She admitted they were, uh, fooling around when Bob lost control of the truck. She had her head in his lap, uh, servicing him, if you know what I mean."

I laughed. "Oh, that's why he didn't have any pants on. I thought the medics cut them off."

"Well, that's not the best part. Another woman shows up earlier this morning, and *she* claims to be Bob's wife. Next thing I know, I get called to the ICU waiting room to find the WWF match of the century. These two gals were in the midst of a serious cat fight, and they both ended up in the ER with black eyes. We had to call the sheriff's office to keep them apart." Diana giggled. "Who do you think is gonna be in big trouble when he wakes up?"

"Guess that would be Bob, Bob, Bob, Bob."

Friday nights often brought us a little entertainment, too. The boys would be out drinking, and we'd often find ourselves dragged out of bed to pick up some drunk who had gotten himself into a barroom brawl.

At least this time it was a beautiful night. The view of the harvest moon rising behind Mount Diablo was spectacular as we headed out for a stab wound to the abdomen. "Base, CAL-STAR One. Lifting at 01:33, en route to Oakley with an ETA of 01:45. Ready to copy map coordinates and frequencies."

"Map coordinates are Thomas Brothers page 26 B4. You'll be talking with Captain 52 on Tac 5. John Muir is open and willing to accept. Be advised you'll be landing in a parking lot near a bar, and the scene is not yet secure."

Our pilot that night was Carl, a marvelous flyer who also happens to be built like a Greek god. The flashing beacons of the emergency vehicles made his navigation to the scene easy; we could see them as soon as we passed over Kirker Pass, some fifteen miles from Oakley. We made radio contact with the fire department, who briefed us on the landing zone and brought us down uneventfully in the parking lot next to the Come Back Inn, a bar notorious for the hard-drinking crowd it lured. On weekends it featured some local band that played behind chicken wire to protect them from the beer bottles the crowd frequently hurled toward the stage. Crowds of bar patrons milled behind the police lines, obviously entertained by the activity we created. As I walked through the parking lot to the ambulance, several of the men started yelling, "Hey, nursie, nursie! I need help!" as they fell to the ground laughing and clutching their chests. I grinned at their antics as I opened the back door of the ambulance.

I was greeted by Joe, a paramedic I had met years before when I was his preceptor during his emergency room training. "Hey Janice, how you doing?" he asked, planting a chaste kiss on my cheek.

"I was sleeping soundly, thank you, before you guys got us involved. What do you have for us tonight?" I surveyed the rather pasty-looking patient lying on the gurney.

"Well, seems José here was enjoying a night on the town and he had an unfortunate misunderstanding with another patron. He was stabbed, once in the right upper quadrant. It's bleeding quite a bit."

I reached over and lifted up the blood-soaked dressing that covered the wound. "Any bowel protruding?" I asked. Blood spurted from an artery and barely missed my face. I slapped it down hastily. "Jeez, you weren't kidding. That's pretty impressive." Judging from his skin signs and barely palpable pulse, José was about to get a whole lot sicker if we couldn't get him to the OR to get the bleeding controlled.

"José," I yelled into our patient's ear. "We're going to fly you to the trauma center, OK? Where do you hurt the most?"

José peered at me through a drunken haze, trying to focus on my face. "Hey, I got stabbed. My stomach hurts."

Having thus cleverly established that José had an intact airway and adequate blood pressure, I stepped back to get the big picture. Our friend was lying on the stretcher, wearing only a pair of boxer shorts cheerfully printed with large red hearts, albeit now soaked with blood. His hair was carefully slicked back and combed into a swirl. An overwhelming odor of cheap cologne and tequila hung in the air. Clearly this man was out on the prowl tonight. But the most impressive addition to his ensemble was a pair of the shiniest black patent leather shoes I had ever seen. Here was a man who took his recreation seriously.

"Hey, José," I said. "Those are some great shoes you got."

His eyes lit up and he wiggled his toes as he regarded his prized possessions. "Yeah. I just got them today."

One of the firefighters popped his head into the ambulance to see what was happening. "Hey you guys, check out his shoes," he said. Everyone murmured that they were indeed some of the best shoes they had ever seen. José beamed with pride.

I headed back to the helicopter and tossed the trauma bag onto the seat. Carl was hunched down in his seat, punching numbers into the computer, estimating weight and balance before lift off. "So how much does this guy weigh?" he asked, keying up the mike.

"I'd say about 75 kilograms—and he's got these really great shoes." Carl turned to look at me with a puzzled expression, but had no chance to inquire further, as the firefighters had arrived to load the patient—complete with those shiny shoes sticking out from under the silver Thermadrape. (Ostensibly, the Thermadrape is there to keep the patient warm, but it also keeps him from bleeding all over the floor of the helicopter, which can short out the wiring and is a mess to clean up.) Carl keyed up the intercom and agreed that José was sporting some pretty fine footwear.

Our flight time to John Muir was about eight minutes, during which we were busy placing more large-bore IVs and delivering fluids. José's BP continued to drop from his rather spectacular blood loss. Despite his deteriorating condition, however, occasionally he would crane his head around to check on his beloved shoes.

As we arrived at the helipad, I hurried into the trauma room ahead of our patient to give report; José needed to get to the OR quickly or he would bleed to death. Just as I finished report, a barely conscious José was wheeled into the room, and the trauma surgeon took hold of the patient's ankles in order to move him to the hospital gurney. This doctor would later repair a large liver laceration and save our hero's life. But before getting down to work, he paused to make an observation. "Yo, José," he said. "Where'd you get these great shoes?"

My first clue that this next call was going to be an adventure came when Kirstie, our dispatcher, seemed a little agitated when I picked up the phone.

"Where are we going on this lovely Sunday night?" I asked.

"This is a weird one," she said. "You've been activated to respond to the Ohlone Wilderness Area for a reported mountain lion mauling. Alameda County Sheriff's is on the line with a young woman who sounds hysterical. They're in some trailer out there and she's screaming that her boyfriend is lying on the floor bleeding after being attacked by a mountain lion."

I scratched my head. "You must be joking. There aren't any mountain lions in the Bay Area, at least none I know of. Bobcats, maybe, but mountain lions?"

"I just dispatch helicopters," Kirstie replied. "I don't come up with the stories."

As we lifted off, I relayed the story to the rest of the crew. Ken, one of our newer flight nurses, was enthusiastic. "A mountain lion mauling?" he asked. "Oh God, this job is just too cool. I can't believe I'm getting paid to do this."

J.B. was a bit more skeptical. "A mountain lion attack? Are they nuts?"

"Stranger things have happened," I reminded him, and off we flew into the moonlight, headed for the Ohlone Wilderness. The night was clear and crisp, and I sat back to enjoy a free helicopter ride that probably wouldn't amount to anything. Ken was busy working the radios with his usual enthusiasm, keeping the entire Bay Area EMS and law enforcement system apprised of our progress. As we approached the wilderness area, Ken contacted the fire unit that was en route.

"Engine 1791, this is CALSTAR One. We are currently over the Los Padres Boy Scout Camp overflying Mines Road southbound. We do not yet have you in sight. Please let us know when you have a visual on us."

"CALSTAR One, this is Engine 1791. We're about sixteen miles farther down Mines Road near mile marker thirty-two. We have been advised by county communications that this incident is on Mercer Ranch. We have entered a radio dead zone, so we'd appreciate you relaying information for us. We'll let you know when we have you in sight. Also, could you ascertain who's joining the party tonight? This dispatch seems pretty suspicious, and we'd appreciate having law enforcement backup."

"Engine 1791, CALSTAR One. Read and check. We understand CDF, Regional Ambulance, CHP and Alameda County Sheriff's all responding. Happy to relay for all. We'll be overhead in a few."

Looking back down Mines Road in the direction we had come, I saw a string of flashing red beacons. After a few radio calls, we discovered all the agencies Ken mentioned were responding, and a few more as well. "Must be a pretty quiet night in Livermore to get this kind of response," I thought aloud. "Must be half of the law enforcement and EMS personnel on duty in a fifty-mile radius down there. Probably a few off-duty officers as well."

"Well, this is really starting to be quite the party," J.B. added.

After a few minutes, we spotted Engine 1791, which was stopped at the side of the road. J.B. initiated a high orbit, as the firefighters decided to wait for the rest of the party to catch up. They would be turning onto an unmarked dirt road that the others might easily miss. The dirt road stretched on for miles, so we decided to contact Alameda County Sheriff's Office—or Alco—to see if the woman who made the call could be more helpful about where this trailer might be.

"Alco, this is CALSTAR One. We're currently over Engine 1791 on Mines Road at approximately the fifty-three-mile marker, where the turnoff to Mercer Ranch is located. Can you recontact the reporting party for instructions as to their specific location? The rest of the group should be here in approximately ten minutes."

"CALSTAR One, this is Alco. Be advised we have the woman back on the telephone. We are having great difficulty in gaining any information from her. She is hysterical and will not cooperate with us. We are hearing sounds of multiple gunshots in the background. We are unsure what type of situation we are dealing with. We'll try and get more specific directions. Understand all units are in a radio dead zone, and you will be relaying all information."

"That's affirm for CALSTAR One. We'll stand by till you can get further instructions to us."

"Hey J.B.," I said. "Could we get a couple of thousand feet up? As you know, we look suspiciously like a police helicopter, and I suspect these people are not real rational."

"Yeah, that seems to be the prudent thing to do," he replied. "You know, I think I'm catching a whiff of bullshit here."

The ambulance, fire engines and the first police cars had now assembled below us, and they all turned onto the rutted dirt road, leaving a strobe light to mark the turnoff for the others following. In the moonlight we could see the huge fire engine groaning over the deeply rutted surface, making the going rather slow. We decided to fly ahead and try to locate the trailer ourselves and guide the party in, keeping a distance from the madness below.

Alco contacted us with an update. "CALSTAR One, this is Alco. The reporting party is back on the line. She now states they are being *overrun* with mountain lions—they are reportedly surrounding the house and attacking. We continue to hear gunshots being fired."

Oh, jeez. "Alco, we copy you 10-2. Overrun with mountain lions. Be advised we are reluctant to approach the scene without the benefit of law enforcement, and will commence a high orbit."

"CALSTAR One, Alco. We concur with high orbit until the sheriff is on scene. Oh, and by the way, the woman now states there must be forty or fifty lions attacking them."

About fifteen minutes later, the first fire engine reached the trailer and Engine 1791 came up on the radio. We could hear a screaming, incoherent woman in the background. "CALSTAR, we are on scene. As suspected, there are no mountain lions in the vicinity, and no injuries. There are, however, four very intoxicated individuals and one very frightened, pregnant house cat. There are multiple shotgun holes in the trailer. All medical personnel can be released. Law enforcement to continue in. Thanks for coming tonight."

The story made the front page in the *Livermore Times*. It seems two young men had taken their underage girlfriends out to the hills and had broken into a trailer on a remote ranch. They had thoughtfully provided a great deal of alcohol and methamphetamine—crystal meth—which they had been delving into deeply for two days. In a drunken, drug-induced frenzy, they had mistaken the pregnant cat for a mountain lion, and the hallucination escalated from there.

The young men were taken to jail, and the girls were taken home to their parents. The family that owned the trailer put new locks on the door. The cat was taken to the SPCA for the duration of her confinement.

CHAPTER EIGHT

Why I Missed Vince's Party

"LADIES and gentlemen, welcome to the 1989 World Series, brought to you by KNBR radio. I'm Ron Fairly, and we're coming at you live from Candlestick Park for the third game between the San Francisco Giants and the Oakland A's. This Bay Bridge series is the most exciting sporting event of the decade. Bill, why don't you get us up to speed on the series thus far?"

"Well, Ron..." Static on our cheesy AM radio obscured Bill's response. I glanced at the clock; it was only 4:50 p.m. My shift in the emergency room at Seton would be over at 5:30, and quitting time couldn't come early enough. The day had been long and tedious, filled with surly patients and uncooperative families. I knew the department would be busy after the game, as alcohol-fueled baseball fans descended on the city. I was pleased to know I would not have to be involved in that hootenanny. I was scheduled the following day for a shift at CALSTAR and would be safely tucked into my own bed long before the drunks landed in the ER.

Since we had a lull, I wandered out through the ambulance doors into a spectacular October afternoon. As I sat down against the wall, turning my face to the warm sun, I wondered if I should try and brave the traffic to get to Vince's World Series party in Berkeley that evening. It meant driving across the Bay Bridge during rush hour traffic. Vince Scott, one of the ER docs and a famed cook, was throwing a bash at his house. Inside, he was hustling to get his charts done quickly so he could zoom home before the rest of his guests arrived. His roommate had called several times during the afternoon with minor crises, the last of which was a spinach soufflé that refused to rise. "We'll just call it a terrain," an exasperated Vince had yelled into the phone. "Don't worry about it. Worst comes to worst, we'll go to 7-Eleven and get some chips and dip." I glanced down at my watch. It was now 4:55, and I looked up to see Vince running out toward his rusty blue pickup truck.

As he threw his briefcase onto the passenger seat, he looked back at me basking in the sun. "So are you coming tonight?" he asked.

"Of course," I said, "except the traffic is going to be a nightmare."

"I know," he said. "I'm on my way now. Maybe everybody in the greater Bay Area will be at the game, or at least watching it. I have a house full of guests, and my roommate is going nuts. Anyway, you have directions. Call if you get lost."

"Thanks, Vince. I'm off at 5:30, so it'll be after six when I get there. Is it OK if I wear my scrubs? I didn't bring a change of clothes with me."

"Janice, you're welcome to wear anything you want." He hopped into the truck and wheeled out of the parking lot, waving.

I wandered back inside and found Bob, the ER doc who had taken over from Vince, writing in a chart. "Oh, Janice," he said, "I was just looking for you. Can you set up a suture tray with 4-0 nylon in 4B? The guy fell through a plate-glass window at work and has a pretty deep laceration in his thigh. Come to think of it, open two sutures for me, OK?"

"Bob, for you, the world," I replied. "Hey, how did you manage to draw the short straw to be on tonight?" I asked.

"I missed the last staff meeting, and I got elected," he said, grinning. "That'll teach me, huh?"

I picked up the supplies and headed to room 4B, where I introduced myself to a young man sitting quietly and holding a very bloody dressing over his wound. I got the sutures ready and Bob wandered in a minute later. "You ready to get started, sport?" he asked the patient.

"Ready as I'll ever be." He turned his head away gritting his teeth as Bob began to infiltrate the wound with local anesthetic.

I wandered back to the nursing station, got a glass of water, and sat down next to Mary Janet, a fellow nurse. In the background, the pre-game radio show was still in progress. "So are you going to Vince's party?" she asked as I made a note on a chart.

"I think so. It's not every day the World Series features our own teams, and I'm sure the food is going to be fabulous."

"Wish I could go," M.J. said moodily. "But I'm here till ten o'clock. Just about the time all hell breaks loose."

"Don't worry, I'll eat enough for two, OK?" She grinned and returned to her charting.

"Hey, what was that?" she asked suddenly. I looked down and noticed the water in my cup sloshing over the rim. Then everything around us began to rattle. We both looked up at the same time and then heard a loud growling rumble as the walls began to shake.

"I think we're having an earthquake, that's what," I said, standing up unsteadily, as the floor was now beginning to pitch and sway. Realizing the nursing station was surrounded by glass walls, we both began moving toward the ambulance doors. As we were standing up, Bob came running down the hall, headed for the parking lot with his patient right behind him, the unfinished suture streaming from his thigh and dripping blood. As we reached the doorway, the shaking became more intense. I watched the asphalt move in a slow undulating wave, and nearby a forty-foot pine tree thrashed violently back and forth. The noise became a crescendo of booming thunder as the earth beneath us shifted. After what seemed like forever, the waves slowed and the rumble died out. We all stood uneasily for a moment and stared at one another, unsure if Mother Nature was really finished.

Bob broke the silence. "Well, that was a pretty good shaker. Must have been at least a four or five." The emergency generator in the corner of the parking lot kicked in, spewing diesel fumes into the air.

We moved back into the ER, now joking and laughing. Edita, our unit clerk, set up a pool on the size of the earthquake. "Put me down for five bucks on a 5.3," I said, handing over the cash.

"Aw, you're crazy," M.J. said, handing Edita another five dollars. "That was a 6.0 if I've ever seen one." Everyone else crowded around, handing over their bets as Edita furiously scribbled down the various guesses. (We would learn later that the earthquake was in fact a 7.1.) In the nursing station, several books had been knocked off the shelf, but no other damage was apparent. In the background, KNBR continued its coverage of the baseball game, and the commentators were busy setting up their own betting pool.

"Well, everybody seems to be OK here at Candlestick," the

announcer said. "The players and fans are milling around. I don't see any damage to the park, but they have the engineers out here to check on everything before we get into the game. Boy, oh, boy, this is an unprecedented addition to an already historic World Series. First we have the two Bay Area rivals playing, and now we have an earthquake to boot! Don't worry, folks, looks like all's well here."

"Well, Ron, this sure is a historic moment—" Bill was abruptly cut off by the emergency broadcasting system's attention signal: "Regular broadcasting has been interrupted because of an imminent or current disaster state. Please stand by for emergency information."

Silence filled the airwaves. Everyone at the station looked up from what they were doing and stared at the radio. They must be overreacting, I thought. After all, we were all fine, weren't we? Another voice came on the air, a roll call of the Bay Area county EMS dispatchers.

"This is a roll call for Bay Area EMS. San Francisco County?"

"San Francisco present. Communications partially intact. Unknown extent of damage."

"Alameda County?"

"Alameda County present, communications mostly disrupted, initial report of a partial freeway collapse."

"San Mateo County?"

"San Mateo County present, reports unclear. Initial report of multiple damaged structures, extent unknown. Communications partially disrupted."

"Santa Clara County?"

Silence, followed by another query. "Santa Clara County, please respond." Silence. "Santa Clara County, this is the Bay Area Emergency Network. Please respond." In the background, we heard a terrified voice. "We can't raise Santa Clara, we can't raise Santa Clara!" The broadcast was abruptly cut off by ominous static.

At that moment, the medics ran in. Their previously jovial expressions were now replaced with deep concern. "We've been monitoring county dispatch. This one is bad. The Amfac hotel at the airport has collapsed, there's a huge fire in the Marina district of San Francisco, and a portion of the Bay Bridge has collapsed. This thing is gonna get real bad, real fast. You guys better implement your disaster plan and get some people in here now."

The enormity of this earthquake was only starting to sink in—this was no garden variety Bay Area shaker. Suddenly it didn't seem like so much fun. Just then the double doors to the registration area burst open, and a man came rushing in carrying a woman with two broken femurs. "I need some help," he screamed in panic. "A wall fell down on her and broke both her legs." Susan, M.J. and I scrambled for a gurney, and they wheeled the patient back to the ortho room, which now had no lights. I glanced out of the ambulance doors and looked north toward San Francisco. Huge columns of black smoke billowed up from the Marina district, and the wailing of sirens was everywhere. Things were starting to happen quickly.

Susan, who had the unenviable job of charge nurse that night, returned from the ortho room and pulled out the disaster manual, frantically trying to locate the earthquake section. She pulled out policy after policy, all of which were absolutely useless. Only the emergency lights were available in the back room. M.J. had found several flashlights, and two of the techs were holding them for the orthopedists as they struggled in the gloom to treat the woman with the broken femurs. We might as well have been treating her in somebody's basement. I stood for a few minutes watching the eerie scene.

Mark was working in the ICU that night and I decided that when I had a moment I would go over to check on him. But for now, we had to get the emergency triage center set up. I walked back to the nursing station and found Susan still desperately flipping through the policy and procedure manuals. Thankfully, David Goldschmid, our ER director, ran in through the doors. "What's happening?" he asked as he pulled off his coat.

"The hospital seems to be OK, but we only have generator power," Susan told him. "We have got one critical patient—a woman who broke both femurs. Ortho is with her right now with M.J. I can't find the earthquake disaster policy. Do you know where it is?"

He shook his head. "We've been reworking that one. So this is how we're going to start: Assign at least one nurse to each of the critical care rooms. I'm going to set up a rapid triage table outside in the waiting room, and get Bob and another nurse to man that. They can manage all the minors, and we'll have them ship back anyone who's serious. Janice, you get on the phone and try to find out the status of both CALSTAR and Stanford Lifeflight in case we need to get anyone out. Then start calling all the staff, both doctors and nurses, and ask them to come in if they can. We need as many people as possible. Susan, call the nursing office and the OR to find out bed and staff availability. Then call the county and let them know how many casualties we can take. In the meantime, I'll help Bob set up triage outside."

Suddenly I remembered Vince's party. "David, Vince just left here twenty minutes ago. He might have been on the Bay Bridge when it collapsed."

David grew pale. "The Bay Bridge collapsed? I hadn't heard that yet." We all stopped and stared at one another until David spoke. "We can't do anything about that right now. Janice, try the staff in the immediate area first, then try to call his house. Maybe he was already home. Let me know either way, OK?"

I headed for the phone, glad to have something to keep me busy. I grabbed the employee phone list and began, but with each call I was met with, "Please try your number later. All circuits are busy." Methodically, I continued to dial each person on the list, and each time got the same frustrating message. I dialed Vince's house three times and was unable to get through. My increasing panic was interrupted by Susan.

"Janice, we need you out here now," she hollered as she pushed a man clutching his chest past the nursing station into one of the critical care rooms. He was gray, diaphoretic, and seemed to be having a hard time breathing. I dropped the phone and followed them into room 2, helping Susan undress our patient as she gave me his story.

"This is Mr. Flanagan. He had a sudden onset of severe crushing chest pain right after the earthquake," she said as she hoisted him up to the bed. "I'll help you get started, but the waiting room is starting to fill up."

"Just go get me the twelve-lead EKG, then go ahead back out. But send David in here on your way out, OK?" I nodded reassuringly to our patient.

"So, Mr. Flanagan, having a little excitement here today," I said as I hooked him up to the EKG. His EKG confirmed what we had already suspected: he was indeed having a very large, possibly lethal heart attack. The monitor displayed a pattern we call tombstones—a fitting name, because this is a grave clinical indicator. His blood pressure was quite low, and his oxygen saturation was on the downhill slide, indicating fluid was starting to back up into his lungs from his failing heart.

I placed him on high-flow oxygen, started an IV, and

obtained the blood work we needed before starting TPA, the "clot-busting drug." David had come in and was looking over my shoulder as the machine spit out the EKG results. I glanced at him as he picked it up, and he nodded. "TPA," was all he said, and then returned to the station. While I was working, I picked up the phone and dialed the nursing supervisor, with my back to the patient so he couldn't hear me. "Claudette, got a Mr. Flanagan here with a big anterior wall MI. We're gonna need an ICU bed, and he might need to go to the cardiac cath lab. Nothing official yet, just wanted to give you a heads-up."

"Thanks, Janice," she said, "I'll keep a bed open in the coronary care unit. Let me know when he's officially admitted and whether we have to call the cath lab team in."

"Will do," I said, and stuck my head out of the room to get David's attention. He was juggling two phones and trying to write at the same time. "Hey David, are we going to take him to the cath lab or do TPA here?"

"Dr. Brown is on his way up to see him now," he said, "I think he wants to take him downstairs to the lab for intracoronary TPA. But get everything ready to go here." I started to draw up the medication.

As I was working, Mark wandered in from the ICU. "What are you guys up to?" he said, giving me a peck on the cheek. He glanced at the monitor and softly whispered in my ear, "Jesus—that's pretty impressive." I nodded, relieved to see him and know he was all right.

"We're a little busy here, getting ready to go down to the cath lab. Mr. Flanagan, this is Mark Hudson. He's a nurse over in the ICU, and happens to be my husband."

Mr. Flanagan held up a shaky hand to Mark. "Pleased to meet ya," he said. "You'll have to excuse me. I'm not feeling so good."

I looked back at Mark. "Could you do me a favor? Go to the nursing station and get me ten milligrams of morphine. We have to try and get rid of some of his chest pain, and I've got to get a dopamine drip started for his blood pressure." Mark nodded and trotted off to the station. I turned to Mr. Flanagan. "You sure picked quite a day to get sick. First the World Series, now an earthquake."

Mark returned to the room with the morphine. I gestured for him to give it. "Start with two milligrams. He's still hypotensive, and the dopamine hasn't kicked in yet. So how did you all fare in the ICU?"

"It's not too bad now," he said. "Want a second IV?" I indicated yes, and he set up his equipment as we talked. "When everything started shaking, we all dove under the console desk, and when it was all over, every monitor in the joint had heart rates over 150. We ran around and gave everybody Valium and a couple of people Adenosine, and got everything settled down. One guy was really upset. He figured he had given up smoking, drinking, lost fifty pounds and had taken up jogging, and still landed in the OR for a coronary bypass. Then we have an earthquake, and he's convinced we're all gonna die. I had to assure him that the hospital was not going to come crashing down. Of course, a little Valium and some morphine helped." He turned to Mr. Flanagan. "Is the chest pain any better?"

"A little," Mr. Flanagan replied. "Ya know, I feel kind of the same way."

Half an hour later, I had Mr. Flanagan down in the cardiac catherization laboratory, where they run tests to see which coronary arteries are blocked, and possibly try to clear them. When I returned to the ER, I found the nursing station crawling with bodies—administrative suit-type bodies. The ER staff was busy trying to manage the hoards of mostly minor injuries that had flooded the department, but were having difficulty navigating through the crush of suits, who were making mysterious notes on clipboards. His Highness the CEO had arrived and was surrounded by nervous aides who scrambled after him as he moved from spot to spot, furiously taking notes as he spoke. I ran into Susan, who was running down the hallway carrying an armload of charts. "What's going on here?" I asked. "I can't even get into the station to get meds because of all the bodies. What are they doing here?"

"I know, I know. David keeps chasing them out, but they keep coming back." She handed me a couple of charts.

Outside the doors, an ambulance pulled up with a screech. As they pulled the patient out of the rig, we could clearly hear him yelling. "God damn it! God damn it! I can't believe this shit!" Susan looked at me, shrugged, and took the charts back.

"Room 12," she said to the ambulance crew, and headed off.

As the medics wheeled our distraught patient into the room, they gave me a brief report. "This gentleman was in one of the luxury boxes at Candlestick. After the earthquake, he started having chest pain. So here he is. We have to get back there—lots of patients lining up at the first aid station. We'll get the paperwork back to you later."

"Fine," I said as I turned my attention to our obviously distraught patient, who seemed to be close to tears. He clutched my arm, babbling as I tried to take off his shirt and hook him up to the monitors.

"All my life I've been waiting for this day," he ranted. "My son, my oldest son, is playing in the World Series. I flew in from Miami this morning—had a huge party last night. And the day I get to see my own son playing in the World Series, there's an earthquake! A goddamn earthquake! All my life I've been waiting for this, I tell you! And now I'm having a goddamn heart attack! It's not fair. I mean I coached this kid from the time he was in diapers, always praying for this day. And now I'm never gonna see him play again, 'cause I'm gonna die from a frickin' heart attack." While he was raving, I pulled off his shirt and placed him on the cardiac monitor. Sure enough, he was having a large heart attack.

I tried to calm him down a bit. "We're not going to let you die," I said in my most reassuring tone. I asked him his son's name but, being only a fair-weather baseball fan, I didn't recognize it.

"I'll be right back," I said to him. "I'm going to get some medicine for your pain and have the doctor take a look at you. Your job right now is to try and relax. All of this screaming isn't helping your heart."

I hurried back to the station, pushing my way through the expanding crowd of suits. "I need one of the docs for another MI in 12," I yelled over the din, to no one in particular. "Anybody around?" I scanned the crowd, looking for a doctor. To my delight, Vince came striding through the door, pulling on his lab coat.

"Oh my God, Vince," I said, hugging him tightly. "Where were you? We were afraid that you were on the bridge when it collapsed. Are you all right?"

"I'm fine," he said, hugging me back. "Little shook up, but OK. And yes, I was on the bridge. Mid-span right before Treasure Island. I was listening to the radio, when my truck started shaking. At first I thought all four tires blew out at the same time, then I realized everybody around me was having a problem, too. Then everything stopped. When we figured out what had happened, every car on that bridge was trying to turn around and get off as quick as they could. It was mayhem. I was afraid there was going to be an aftershock and the whole bridge would go. There was no way I was going to get home, so I came back here. Figured you all might need some help." He glanced around at the chaos. "Looks like I made the right decision."

"We were so worried about you. And yes, you did make the right decision," I said, propelling him toward room 12. "I have a patient in need of your services at this very moment." I pushed Vince into the room and introduced him to our patient. "He was watching his son play in the World Series when the earthquake started. Sitting in one of those fancy luxury boxes. Now he's having a lot of chest pain." I pushed the twelve-lead EKG under his nose.

"Yes, I believe he is having that heart attack," he said. This was the fourth MI in our department within two hours.

Things in the rest of the department were starting to get under control. David had finally escorted the administrators to another command post, where they set up what they called "the nerve center," whatever that was. Ten off-duty nurses showed up of their own accord, along with almost as many physicians. Every room was staffed with two nurses and one doctor, and a fast-track clinic was up and running to manage the flood of patients with minor bumps and bruises. With all the help we were catching up.

My thoughts turned to my family. I knew they would be watching the Series, and through the magic of television there probably wasn't a human being in the developed world unaware of the events in San Francisco that night. Most of the television stations were beaming out live clips of the Marina burning, and of the Cypress Freeway in Oakland that had collapsed, killing most of the unlucky souls trapped on the lower deck. But despite the intense damage in isolated spots, the Bay Area had dodged the bullet again. This was not the Big One. Unfortunately, most of the country didn't know that. From the horrific pictures, it appeared that San Francisco had fallen into the ocean or was at least going to burn to the ground.

I knew my family would be frantic. Repeatedly I dialed for an outside line, only to be met with that irritating message: "Please try your call again later. All circuits are busy." Finally, after a half-hour of diligent dialing, I made it through. Of course, their phone was busy. "When are they going to get call waiting?" I thought angrily as I tried again and again. I was to learn later they were on the phone with my sister, who then lived in St. Louis. Together they were busy worrying about Mark and me, unaware I was trying to get through. Finally, I had an operator break through the line with an emergency call.

At nine o'clock, I was finally released to go home. I had no idea what would be waiting at our little condo in Brisbane. To my surprise, the power was on and the outside of the building didn't appear to be damaged. I ran up the steps two at a time and stood uncertainly at the front door, afraid to open it. Taking a deep breath, I unlocked the door and it swung open. Roscoe flung himself into my arms, shaking and crying, but unhurt. I flipped on the lights. Aside from the artwork hanging a bit askew and a few books knocked off the bookcase, nothing was damaged. It was all very strange, and the strangeness persisted for days.

While we had been struggling in the Seton emergency department, another story was unfolding at CALSTAR.

Andy was in the hangar setting up chairs for a class that evening, while Rose and Tim were upstairs watching the pre-game blather. As the earthquake began, the hangar door began to shake, and as Andy ran outside, he saw the ground pitch, rocking his truck two or three feet back and forth. Beyond the parking lot, the airport runways appeared to be moving in waves.

When the shaking subsided, Tim and Rose ran downstairs to check for damage. The helicopter had been rocked, too, but not damaged. Because the phones and electricity were out, and therefore probably the pagers as well, they realized that dispatch had no way to contact them except by radio. Anyway, with the phones down, it would be impossible for county agencies to contact CALSTAR dispatch.

The crew piled into the helicopter and cranked up the radios. There was general bedlam on all of the county channels. At one point the Alameda County Emergency Channel (CMED) dispatched four ambulances to a "building collapse" on Cypress Street in Oakland. Andy keyed up the mike and asked if they wanted CALSTAR to respond, to which he received an enthusiastic affirmative.

As they approached the area where the building had reportedly collapsed, they could see smoke rising from the Cypress Freeway, a double-decker viaduct in downtown Oakland. The structure looked odd—it appeared to have melted into a ribbon of asphalt and concrete. As usual, the initial reports were inaccurate: It was not a building that had collapsed, but rather a long section of this freeway. The top section had caved in, crushing everything on the lower deck beneath tons of concrete and rubble.

The crew watched in horror as people swarmed out of their cars, trying to escape, while others below gestured wildly at the helicopter, asking them to land and render assistance. Only ten or twelve minutes had elapsed since the earthquake had rumbled through.

Andy relayed to CMED what they were witnessing, which was probably the first accurate description of the earthquake's most lethal result. Tim began to orbit lower, considering landing on the partially collapsed structure. But when they were twenty or thirty feet from the surface, they all decided it was too dangerous. For all they knew, the additional weight of the helicopter might be enough to send the whole thing crashing to the ground. They veered back into the sky, trying to decide on a course of action.

The main problem was that they could not communicate with any of the firefighters below; no central radio frequency had been assigned. By this time the CHP helicopter had arrived, and both decided to set down at a secure helipad at the nearby Oakland Army Base until the fire department could establish a safe LZ. They spent twenty minutes at the base treating civilians for minor injuries, the most serious of which was a woman whose bookshelf had fallen on her head.

At last, both helicopters were assigned an LZ on West Grand Avenue, adjacent to the Cypress structure. The scene still was not under control. As CALSTAR was on short final, a car raced directly through the LZ, though once it was shooed off they landed uneventfully. A paramedic directed them to an extrication in progress down the street—a truck on the upper deck had been violently thrown off the structure, landing thirty feet below.

EMS personnel and firefighters were swarming over the freeway, looking for survivors. Neighbors came by with ladders and attempted to help anyone who might still be alive on the lower deck, or get people off the upper deck. The fire department was methodically moving down the freeway, peering into the lower deck, which now only afforded a foot or two of space, marking "DOA" in black spray paint whenever a body was discovered. Unfortunately, there were only a few survivors on that level. Almost everyone trapped in the collapse was fatally crushed.

When CALSTAR's patient was finally pulled out of his truck, the crew saw he had pulverized the left half of his body.

They worked quickly to get him packaged, and loaded him onto the helicopter. On the way to John Muir, Andy overheard CMED estimate the casualties: 250 dead, 250 critically injured. As it turned out, these numbers were wildly inflated—67 people died in the quake, 42 of whom were on the Cypress Freeway.

After dropping off their patient at John Muir and making two more routine flights, the crew got back to quarters at 2:00 a.m. By that time CALSTAR had a generator for power, and the phones were again working. Once they received word that their homes and families were OK, they finally got several hours of sleep.

Several months later an EMS journal published a picture of Rose yelling for Andy to bring another IV bag for their patient at the Cypress Freeway. Her expression is one of intense concentration, mingled with the fear and horror of what they were witnessing. This picture rekindles all the painful memories of that night. I have a copy of the magazine, but keep it buried deep in a file of old news clippings. I don't look at it often; it's too distressing. And this wasn't *the* earthquake that is coming, according to those who know about such things. I'm not sure I want to know what that will bring.

CHAPTER NINE

Too Close to Home

I was the type of prepubescent girl who forever pestered mom and dad for a pony. I had horse posters, a zillion horse models, and bookshelves filled with horse stories, of which Black Beauty was my favorite. When I got into my teens, my folks finally relented and allowed me to lease a beat-up school horse, probably in an effort to keep me out of trouble, or at least to shut me up. My first horse was an old swaybacked creature named Carou, whom I loved desperately. He was absolutely bulletproof and remarkably forgiving. We could have hung from his nose and he wouldn't have minded. A year later, I moved up to a monstrous Appaloosa gelding named Ulysses, then finally a trim black mare, Targa. These horses patiently taught me how to care for them and how to ride. As I got into high school, boys and parties began to consume my interest and horses gradually faded from the immediate picture. But I never lost that passion.

Recently I rekindled that old romance. Istanbul Mogul, known as Stanley to those of us who know and love him, was a retired race-horse who belonged to a friend, Liz. In his day he was fairly suc-cessful on the California circuit until he broke his leg on the racetrack, got a plate put into his ankle and was retired. Liz bought him and turned him into a pasture horse. So he was left to his own devices for some fifteen years. Several people tried to take him on, but they considered him too old and lame. Everyone on the ranch knew him, both because of his sweet temperament and his enor-mous size, but no one thought he was more than an amiable lawn ornament.

I met Stanley in 1999, when Liz offered to let me go out and ride him occasionally. In the intervening six months, I started seeing him daily, riding in all weather, training him and slowly building him back up. Gradually, the real Stanley began to emerge—a per-fectly conformed Thoroughbred. Sure, he has arthritis and can't jump fences. On cold mornings he is stiff and I have a hard time keeping weight on him. But everyone who knows him is amazed by the transformation, myself included. We have developed a deep bond and have learned to trust one another.

The following summer, Liz called to tell me she was giving him to me. She understood how much I loved him and wanted us to be together. So Stanley is now family. Mark is still adjusting.

"Good heavens, what happened to you?" I asked, surveying Fred's ankle fracture as the medics rolled him through the emer-gency department and toward the orthopedic room.

"Got my foot caught in the stirrup when a horse threw me, then he dragged me for a ways," Fred replied, grimacing with pain. He held his leg still with both hands, as every tiny move-ment made the muscles spasm. The medics had kindly given him a great deal of morphine en route to the hospital from Half

Moon Bay, but he was still obviously uncomfortable.

"Well, you certainly did a fine job of it," I said. "OK, let's gently lift him over to the gurney. On three. One, two, three." Gently, we moved him to the bed. He was covered with dirt, and his injured ankle was still in a mud-caked riding boot bent inward at an unnatural angle. "Does your neck or anything else hurt? Did you pass out or hit your head?" I asked as I started helping him get undressed.

"I think I pulled a couple of muscles in my back when I got dragged, but everything else is OK," he replied through gritted teeth. "I need to use the phone," he added. "I have to make sure the horses got put away."

"You can do that as soon as I get you settled in," I said. "So what happened?"

"I'm the caretaker of a quarter-horse ranch down in Half Moon Bay. I was out riding on one of the mares who doesn't like water. When I made her walk past a puddle she spooked and bolted. She reared up, I fell off, and my foot was still in the stirrup. Got dragged about a hundred feet down the trail through the mud until she stopped."

"Is she always that bad?"

"She has her moments." He winced as I pulled off his clothes.

While I helped him into a patient gown, I pushed the gurney over to the phone. "You go ahead and call to check on the horses. I'm going to get some more morphine and get the doc to take a look at this. It's going to hurt a lot when we take that boot off. I can take the edge off with the morphine, but you're going to have to hang in there with us, OK?" He nodded.

Twenty milligrams of morphine later we had the boot off, and I was preparing Fred for surgery. The X-ray revealed a rather impressive ankle fracture that would require an operation to place a plate and screws to stabilize the bones. As I was finishing his paperwork, we started chatting about horses. Fred's employer was an absentee owner who only showed up once or twice a year—someone who liked to say he owned a horse ranch out in California but was really uninterested in the whole affair. Fred cared for seven horses by himself, and lived in a small cottage behind the main house.

"It's not as great as you think it might be," he said. "The horses don't get ridden nearly enough. It's all I can do to just keep the place running and the stalls mucked out. Take Jake, for instance. He's a purebred quarter horse, a former champion barrel racer. He should be worked every day. But I don't have time to ride him. It's a waste."

"Jeez, I'd *love* to have a horse like that," I said. "I'd do almost anything to get to ride regularly again."

"Are you serious? If you want to come down and help me exercise the horses, it would really help me out a lot. Especially now. I don't think I'll be riding for a while with this ankle," he said ruefully.

"I'd love to. Just tell me how soon I can come down, and I'll be there. Like tomorrow?"

Fred laughed. "I think I should probably be there to show you around. OK, this is my offer. You make a commitment to come down at least twice a week, brush two horses and ride one, and we have a deal. What do you say?"

I was thrilled. "Of course. Can Mark, my husband, come along?"

"Does he ride?"

"Used to ride rodeo as a kid in Texas. He's better than I'll ever be."

"Perfect. I'll call you when they let me out of here."

Mark and I went to the ranch a week later, and Fred hobbled around on crutches as he introduced us to the horses. My favorite was Jake, a large black quarter horse gelding with a wonderful disposition. And riding him—what a joy. He was smooth, responsive, and well behaved. He danced as he walked, kicking up his heels just for the fun of it. Fred insisted we stay in the ring until he was well enough to go out on the trail with us, but that was good enough for me.

Fred was grinning as Jake and I loped easily around the ring. "You better watch out, Mark. You're gonna get some competition from that horse. I think I see a love affair starting."

"You're probably right," Mark agreed. "Now she'll never be home."

"And Janice, don't get too attached to ol' Jake there. We've got other horses that need some ring time, too, remember." I knew he was right, but I had already picked my favorite of the bunch.

Several weeks later, Fred was back on his feet, and we planned the big trail ride. Fred was going to be on his own horse, and I finally was going to be able to take Jake out. When I got to the ranch, Fred asked if I would first brush BJ, the horse responsible for breaking his ankle. After I got to know her, it didn't surprise me that she was the one to hurt Fred. She really didn't like people. Every time I went to get her out of her paddock, she would shy away. When I cornered her and got her halter on, she would rush the gate, running me over. When we finally got to the bar to groom her, she would nervously move around, reaching around to bite or step on any available body part. And forget about cleaning out the hooves. She seemed to enjoy taking aim and kicking. If you weren't in kicking range, she'd try to reach around and bite. In short, she was mean, uncooperative and jittery. These are not good characteristics in a horse, particularly considering horses outweigh their riders at least by a factor of ten. I struggled with her for half an hour, and she nearly stomped my instep while I was trying to brush her. I was glad to put her back in her paddock where she couldn't get at me.

Finally it was time for the ride with Jake and I went to collect him. He stood sleepily while I brushed him, and obediently held up his feet for cleaning. While I combed out his mane, he leaned his head on my shoulder and nuzzled my neck. "You are too cute," I whispered to him. When we got to putting the saddle on, he seemed to know that something was different. He began to stir restlessly, anxious to get on with it.

As I suspected, he was fabulous on the trail. We rode for nearly four hours along the rugged San Mateo coastline and ended up at the beach galloping through the surf. It was marvelous—one of those picture-perfect days Madison Avenue would have us believe are real.

Our hobby proved to be a wonderful diversion from the depressing world of medicine. We settled into a routine at the ranch, coming down twice a week to ride. If I could have gotten away with it, I would have just ridden Jake, but the other horses needed to get out as well. One afternoon, Fred asked me to saddle up BJ to take her out. He had been working with her, and wanted me to see if she had made any improvements. Getting her brushed and saddled was a chore, and every time I tried to get on her, she stepped away. When we got out on the trail, it was clear to me nothing had changed. She was spooking at every leaf and noise, and as we were trying to walk through a gate, she balked, then began to rear and buck.

"Don't let up," Fred advised, safe and comfortable on his own horse as BJ bounced in circles. "Just turn her around a couple of times, then walk her through." I was getting increasingly nervous as she became more unruly. "Don't let her get her way. Just keep insisting," he yelled as we spun around. BJ knew she was getting the better of me. Finally, after a dig of my heels, she settled down and nonchalantly walked through the gate.

"Bitch," I muttered under my breath.

Farther down, we encountered a large puddle stretching across the trail. BJ stopped abruptly and refused to walk any far-ther, making it clear to us her aversion to water had not changed. She refused and whirled each time I walked her up to it, becoming more adamant with each attempt. Finally I gave up.

"Fred, we'd better switch horses. I can't get her to do this." Reluctantly he agreed and I dismounted and held her reins. She seemed to know the boss was about to get aboard, and she stood still as Fred climbed up.

"Come on now," he said to her as he turned her back to the puddle. She hesitated, turned several times, then bolted across the puddle, splashing mud all over herself, the saddle, and Fred. "This isn't going to work," he said. "I'm going to see if Niles will work with her. This nonsense has got to stop."

Niles was a handsome young Austrian with a thick accent and a lovely Arabian mare. He was a gifted rider and was known in the area for sorting out problem horses. He had that perfect combination of patience and persistence. Sooner or later, even the densest or the most stubborn horse would get it. Of course, some took longer than others.

BJ continued to be troublesome all the way home, even with Fred in the saddle. By the time we got back to the ranch, she was covered in mud up to her ears, as was the saddle and bridle. Fred took the tack into the barn to clean it and I was left with her, struggling to clean her up. Niles walked into the yard as I was trying, for the fifth time, to get the mud off her nose.

"What's going on?" he asked as we struggled.

"Just being bad again," I said. "Fred had to ride her home."
Fred emerged from the barn, holding the bridle.

"It's that water thing," said Fred. "She just will not walk
through anything wet. She almost threw Janice. I got on her
and made her walk through the puddle, but it wasn't a pretty
picture. This is the result. Got any suggestions?"

"Why is she afraid of the water?" he asked.

"Don't know. She was like that when she got here. I keep
telling the boss to get rid of her, but he won't 'cause of her papers.
Want to take her out tomorrow and see what you can do?".

"Sure," Niles agreed. "I'll take her in the ring first and feel
her out, then we can try a ride. Maybe we need to show her
there's nothing to be afraid of."

They wandered away as they talked. I tried again to brush
BJ's legs, but she wasn't having any part of it. I finally gave up
and sneaked her past Fred when his back was turned. I
quickly unloaded her into the paddock, hoping he wouldn't
notice her legs were still dirty. "Gotta go," I yelled, closing the
gate and beating a hasty retreat to my car.

I was scheduled at CALSTAR the next day, and it turned out to
be beautiful. The sun shone brightly, and a gentle breeze cooled
the hot summer air. The hills were golden brown, and the smell
of barbecues wafted over the airport. Later in the afternoon we
were activated to Half Moon Bay for a drowning.

Most of the time, drowning calls turned out to be dry runs.
Often they were cases of mistaken identity—occasionally the
missing person hadn't even been in the water. If there actually
was a body, the fire department would frequently be unable to
locate it because the powerful tides and currents had washed it
miles away. When that happened, there would be nothing left
to resuscitate. Still, because it was such a lovely afternoon, we

welcomed the helicopter ride to the beach. I was grinning as I keyed up the mike to dispatch.

"CALSTAR Base, CALSTAR One. We have lifted off at 14:48 en route to Half Moon Bay, rough ETA sixteen minutes, getting us there at 15:04. Ready to copy Thomas Brothers map coordinates and radio frequency."

"CALSTAR One, Base. You have been activated for a drowning north of Half Moon Bay, map page 263 B4. Radio frequency will be Half Moon Bay Fire on Calcord, 154.280. Be advised they are unable to locate the victim. Fire department says he may still be immersed. This incident is not on the beach—the victim is reportedly in an irrigation pond east of Highway 1."

"Copy that, Base. Please check availability for Peninsula and Seton Hospitals."

"Base copies. Will do."

I keyed up the intercom. "Doesn't look like this is going to turn into a transport."

Tim agreed. "Yeah, but there are worse things to do on a Sunday afternoon than take a helicopter ride to the coast."

As we cleared the coastal hills heading down to the beach, base called us back. "CALSTAR One, you have been canceled. The body has been located and the patient has expired."

"Well, we're almost there," Tim said. "Want to just fly over the scene to take a gander and then we'll head back home?"

None of us was in any hurry to go back and sit in quarters, so we continued on. As we approached the scene, I realized we were near the ranch. "Hey, you guys, I was just out here yesterday riding. See that barn over there? That's the ranch where I've been spending time. We were just on that trail yesterday."

Tim initiated a high orbit over the irrigation pond where Fred and I had ridden the day before. From our altitude, we could see the paramedics covering a body with a yellow sheet. Several horses standing nearby, restless from all the commotion and the noise of the helicopter, appeared ready to bolt.

"Tim, maybe we better get out of here. We don't want to spook those horses and get somebody else hurt," I said.

"Yeah, you're probably right," he answered and veered off.

When I arrived home the next day, there was a message from Fred on the answering machine. His tone did not relay his usual ebullience. "Call me as soon as you can," was all he said.

I dialed his number, puzzled as to why he sounded so upset. Could he really be that mad at me for putting BJ away without cleaning her legs? Had I left a paddock gate open somewhere?

Fred answered on the third ring. "Fred, it's Janice. I got your message. What's up?"

Fred took a deep breath before answering me. "Janice, there's not going to be any riding around here for a while." I must have done something really horrible to be banned from the ranch. Never again, I vowed, would I ever put a horse away with dirty legs.

"We had a problem out here yesterday. I don't know how to tell you this," he continued. "Niles and BJ were killed." I sank to the floor in disbelief.

"Oh, my God. What happened?"

"Remember how BJ was giving you such a bad time the other day?" he asked. "Well, Niles took her out to try and work with her a bit. We went over to that irrigation pond by the beach." I had the horrible feeling that I knew what he was about to tell me. "Anyway, she wouldn't get into the water. He was making her walk in and out of the water, and she started balking. The next thing I knew, she freaked and plunged into the pond and got her feet tangled underwater. She totally lost it, and started bucking and screaming. At one point, she reared up, and Niles slid off. As he did, she kicked him in the chest and he went under. I ran and jumped to grab him, but she was thrashing around, and I couldn't get to him. Then she went down, too. I swam over to where they had been, but I couldn't find them."

He stopped and sighed heavily. "There were some people going by who had a cellphone, and they called for help. Then they got in the water too and looked for him. But by the time we found him, they had both drowned." A long silence filled the space between us.

"Fred, I was on the helicopter yesterday. We were the ones orbiting overhead. I had no idea it was you and Niles."

"Yeah, I figured that was you. That damn horse. I kept telling the boss to get rid of her, that she was dangerous, but he wouldn't believe me." He sighed again. "Do you want to know the real pisser? If that horse hadn't been so crazy thrashing around like she was, Niles might have gotten away from her. He'd still be alive. When they pulled him out of the water, he had a perfect hoof mark in the middle of his chest. It wasn't a bad enough injury to kill him. He just got the wind knocked out of him and couldn't catch his breath long enough to get away from her while she was thrashing around. By the time we pulled him out, he was gone. They pulled BJ out, too, about an hour later. Her feet were tangled up in old baling wire. Anyway, there's not going to be any riding around here till we get all this straightened out. I hope you understand."

I never did go back to the ranch.

We only flew over the accident that killed Niles and BJ, without having to be involved in the interventions. Later, I had the displeasure of accompanying a colleague on a call that hit even closer to home. We knew it would happen someday.

"CALSTAR One, you have been activated for a scene call to

Highway 1, three miles north of Davenport, for a bicycle accident. How do you copy?"

"Base, CALSTAR One. We copy you 10-2. We have an ETA
of approximately seventeen minutes, getting us there at 13:37.
Ready to copy map coordinates and ground frequency."

Rose and I grinned at each other as we lifted off toward the
coast. She was one of my favorite partners. She's exceptionally
bright and somehow has a smile and a hug for everybody. In
the midst of chaos and tension, Rose always maintains a calm
exterior. She is also acutely aware of the human side of our
care, reminding us these are not simply bodies we are sal-
vaging, but human beings with lives and families. Her perspective calms patients, families and co-workers, and I often
wish I could emulate her style. Unfortunately, if I allow myself
to consider the personal lives of my patients, I can't concentrate on the work at hand. It becomes too painful.

We welcomed this particular flight. The summer weather
was warm and clear, and we had been itching to get out of
quarters on such a lovely day. A helicopter ride out to the spectacular San Mateo coast was a special treat. We didn't expect
the patient to be too critical. More often than not, we were
called not because of the severity of injuries, but because of the
remote location and long transport times.

As we circled the scene, the CDF firefighter began giving us
landing zone instructions. "CALSTAR, we're going to land you on
Highway 1, as there are no appropriate LZs nearby. There is a set of
wires crossing the road a quarter-mile to our north, but no other
obstructions. The wind is negligible. Let us know when you're on
short final, and we'll have CHP shut down traffic." We acknowledged the radio call and scanned the LZ for potential problems. On
my side of the helicopter, I saw our patient lying on a backboard
with the paramedics assisting respirations with a bag-valve mask.

"Uh-oh, Rose. Looks like this isn't going to be a cakewalk after all. I can see the medics bagging him. Doesn't look like he's intubated yet."

"Great," she said. "Get over to me as soon as you can get the helicopter secured, OK?"

"You want me to hold your hand, right?" I teased. She whacked my arm as a reply.

As soon as we landed, I handed her the trauma bag and she scurried off to the patient. I offloaded the litter and took a last look around to ensure the helicopter was secure. To my horror, I saw a reporter and his cameraman running toward the patient, with the helicopter squarely in their path. Clearly intent on getting gory footage for the evening news, they appeared unaware they were about to run directly into our tail rotor. Frantically I waved them off. Aside from the mess they would make if they killed themselves, we already had one patient and we didn't need to add to that number. I glanced over at Rose and the medics. She was lying on her stomach in the gravel trying to intubate the patient. She obviously needed some help, and I was wasting time because of these nitwits.

I ran around the rotor diameter and collared them. "If you come any closer to the helicopter, I'm going to rip your throats out. Get over to the ditch on the side of the road and stay there." They both nodded obediently and sank down into the ditch. I ran over to Rose and the medics who were struggling to secure the patient's airway.

This was not someone who had simply fallen off his bicycle. Half his face was ripped off, and worst of all, one of his eyes stuck out at a crazy angle, dangling by the retinal stalk. He had an open deformity to his chest wall, and through the jagged wound I could see air and blood bubbling out. His trachea was pulled way over to the left, indicating his right lung had collapsed. With every breath he took, more air got trapped in his chest, compressing the good lung and the heart. Because of this crowding in the thorax, his blood pressure was falling dramatically. So was his oxygenation.

Rose was searching for the vocal cords with the laryngoscope. "Got it," she said finally, and slipped the tube into place. I got out the stethoscope and listened for breath sounds. "He's really hard to ventilate," Rose said, and I slapped an air-occlusive dressing over the wound so no more air would get sucked in.

"Rose, I'm only hearing breath sounds on the left. You're going to have to needle his chest."

"I know," she said. "Want to prep him while I get the stuff out?"

I nodded and began to prep his skin with Betadine as she got her equipment ready. "He's got a huge flail segment over here," I said, indicating the multiple rib fractures surrounding the chest wound. Rose nodded and started feeling for her landmarks.

"Yeah, that's the side he was impacted on," she said as she eased the big needle into his chest, releasing the pressure that had built up inside. There was an explosive release of air and blood.

"He's a lot easier to bag now," the medic said.

"Impacted?" I asked. "What happened? I thought he fell off his bicycle."

The medic looked up while he was helping Rose stabilize the pleural needle. "Hit and run. Witnessed by that guy over there," he said, leaning his head toward a small group of people gathered on the other side of the two-lane road. "Car was speeding and veered into this guy, throwing him over forty feet. We found him on the side of the road with his bicycle helmet cracked in half. Driver didn't even stop—just kept on going. He's gotta have some damage to his car. The CHP is looking for his sorry ass right now."

Rose took over bagging the patient as the medics and I finished packaging him. We loaded him into the helicopter as quickly as we could, anxious to get him to the trauma center. As we lifted off, I noted we dusted off the reporters pretty well, much to my satisfaction. Maybe next time they would be a little less intrusive.

Once in the air, Rose began to attach the monitors. I grabbed and arm, looking for an IV. "I HAVE A GREAT ANTE-CUBITAL OVER HERE!" I yelled, not realizing she had switched us to hot mike. "Oops, sorry. Your ears OK? Anyway, you want me to get the IV started?" She nodded, and I began the fluid resuscitation. Meanwhile, Rose gently placed saline-covered gauze over the enucleated eye, protecting it until somebody could put it back where it belonged. I breathed a sigh of relief. Some say the eyes are the windows to the soul, and such a disfiguring injury is unnerving.

We were in the trauma room in fifteen minutes. As we rolled in, the trauma team took over our care with their careful routine. Rose gave report as we handed over care.

"This is a gentleman we estimate to be thirty years old who was struck at freeway speeds out on Highway 1 while on his bicycle—a hit and run. He was wearing a helmet but"—she gestured to remnants of the helmet, lying in pieces between the patient's legs—"you can see it was split in half. He was thrown about forty feet, and was found unresponsive with agonal respirations." She lifted the gauze gently off the eye. "As you can see there is an enucleation, as well as the obvious facial trauma. He also has a large flail segment, and we found him with a tension pneumothorax, with no breath sounds on the left and tracheal deviation. We intubated him, and did a pleural decompression with an immediate improvement of breath sounds and vital signs. There's one large-bore IV on the right; we didn't have time to start a second one." We backed out of the room with our lit-ter and allowed the trauma team to start their work.

I rooted our patient's wallet from his cut and bloodied clothes, retrieved his driver's license and handed the rest of the wallet to the control nurse. "I'll be back with this in a minute so we can get a name and address, OK?" She nodded and I ambled into the break room to start the never-ending ream of paper-work that was generated with each flight. Sitting down heavily, I took a deep breath and stretched. We always became very focused and intense with such a critical patient on board, and I needed a few minutes to decompress before tackling the chart. Rose came clomping into the room, banging the door shut behind her. She was smiling and put her hand up for a high five.

"Eh, how about that?" she said. "What a bitch."

I slapped her hand. "You were fabulous, as always," I said.

She smiled and pulled out a chair, picking up the license. I pulled over the chart, preparing to write the name. "What's his name?" I asked, looking down and ready to copy it onto the front sheet. I heard a choking sound, and looked up. Rose had gone white and was shaking.

"Oh my God, I know this guy," she whispered. She sat down heavily and buried her face in her hands. "He's an artist down in Santa Cruz. He runs a little glass and ceramic shop."

"Oh, Rose. Are you OK?"

She sat quietly for a moment and said, "I have to call Jill, his wife. Where's the phone?"

"Rosie, wait. Maybe there's been some mistake," I said. "Maybe you should go take another look at him before you call her. You better make sure it's really him."

"I don't know if I can look at him right now," she said dully. "But I can't let some stranger call her." She sat quietly for a minute, trying to decide what to do. "Will you come with me?"

I nodded and grabbed her hand. Together we walked back into the trauma room, which had become a very busy place. The surgeons were placing bilateral chest tubes, and general chaos reigned. I spoke quietly to the control nurse. "May we go take a look at this guy again?" I asked. "We think this is a friend of Rose's. She didn't recognize him because of the facial trauma, but it's him on his license."

She put her arm around Rose's shoulders. Together they sidled up to the head of the gurney. Rose looked at him for a minute, dropped her head and cried. "That's him," she said. I followed her as she slowly walked out of the trauma room.

"Do you want me there?" I asked.

"No, I'd rather have some privacy," she said. She walked to the desk and reached for the phone.

The artist died two days later.

High Drama and Low Comedy

FLYING often put us in unusual circumstances and gave us the chance to do some remarkable things.

One day we were activated to the Bay Bridge, which links San Francisco to Oakland. A CHP officer, having just returned from maternity leave, stopped to help the driver of a stalled vehicle on the bridge. While she was standing between the stalled car and her cruiser, the latter was rear-ended by another motorist, pinning her between the cars and fracturing both femurs and her pelvis. An off-duty paramedic supervisor happened on scene and CALSTAR was summoned to transport her to John Muir. The CHP had to close down traffic to allow us to land, and as we were circling, we had the rare opportunity to see the Bay Bridge—usually packed with cars twenty-four hours a day—completely empty. The only other time I saw the bridge devoid of traffic was after the Loma Prieta earthquake of 1989. It's a very strange sight.

It's just as odd to land on an eight-lane freeway to pick up an MVA, and to walk around on a stretch of road that is usually filled with cars whizzing past at seventy miles per hour. That happened fairly frequently when there was a freeway accident and no safe landing zone nearby. The CHP would stop the traffic several hundred feet away from the landing zone, leaving a long line of annoyed motorists. Although we always tried to keep our scene times less than five minutes from skids down to skids up, we hustled a little extra on those calls to help get the traffic moving again.

Another particularly unusual call came on a hot summer day on Mount Diablo, where a man was climbing a formation known as Castle Rock. Our patient had apparently been climbing freehand, with no safety ropes. About halfway up the rock, he lost his grip and tumbled a hundred feet down the face, fracturing his back and both ankles. Because of the remote and inaccessible location, we were first on scene, landing at the top of the rock. We could see him sprawled on the rocks below, surrounded by his climbing companions. Hoisting the trauma bag and packaging gear, we gingerly climbed and slid down to his location. Actually, I bounced down the final ten feet, still clutching the bag and ripping out the seat of my flight suit.

Our patient was awake and writhing in pain. We knew there was no way to haul him back up the way we came without rappelling gear. So we began to cast about for other ways of getting this man off the cliff face as we stabilized and packaged him. The hot sun was radiating off the rocks, and I began to worry about heat stroke—both in the patient and ourselves.

At that point, a winded and red-faced ranger appeared from below as we were placing our patient on the backboard and strapping him in. "You guys aren't going to get him down the way I came," he panted as he reached us. "It's a sheer drop down. We considered our predicament for a few minutes, and then the ranger came up with a plan. "I guess we need to call the Coast Guard helicopter. They have hoisting capabilities."

As it turned out, the Coast Guard was nearby conducting training exercises, and they arrived overhead within ten minutes. It was their massive Sikorsky, and we could hear it approaching from miles away. As this enormous beast hovered overhead, the downwash from its five huge rotor blades was staggering, pushing us to our knees as we covered the patient's face as best we could. The hoist swung out, and the rescue medic was lowered down with a wire Stokes basket, his Neoprene wet suit looking a bit out of place in the hundred-degree heat. As he came down, we helped him unstrap the Stokes, which would be used to transport the patient.

"Unhook that line!" he bellowed, pointing to the extra safety line attached to the hoist. I scrambled over, buffeted by the rotor wash, and unhooked the line. "What happened?" he yelled in my ear.

"He fell about a hundred feet off the rock face, landing on his feet, then his back," I screamed back. His blood pressure is OK, but he's got bad skin signs and he's in a lot of pain."

"OK, let's get him into the Stokes and secured." Together we lifted the backboard and strapped him into the basket. Securing the hoist line and double-checking it, the medic gave an OK sign to the man peering out of the helicopter above us. Slowly our patient began his ascent, sometimes swinging around in a circle. I could only imagine what he must have been thinking.

The medic turned to my partner and me. "Which one of you is the primary nurse?"

"I am," I said. "Why?"

The medic looked up and made another motion to the man in the helicopter. A device that looked like a horse collar appeared at the door and was lowered down to us. "OK," he yelled. "Just put your arms through here and cross them. Remember to keep your arms crossed on the way up, or you'll fall out."

I was stunned. Did this guy think I was actually going to allow myself to get hoisted a hundred feet into thin air, hanging onto that flimsy contraption? Was he nuts? But it was too late. He was already pulling the collar over my head, and the next thing I knew my feet were dangling off the ground. I was pulled up at what seemed like a very rapid rate, leaving me dangling over the sharp rocks below. "Don't look down, don't look down," I whispered to myself, shutting my eyes tightly and gripping the collar for dear life.

The hoist stopped abruptly, and as I opened my eyes, I was just below the hovering helicopter. The winds were whipping me from side to side. "Oh my God, the hoist is stuck," I thought. "And if my arms come uncrossed I will die." A moment of panic ensued, and I took several deep breaths to pull myself together. Then the hoist started moving again slowly, and soon my head was level with the open helicopter door. Two men grabbed my shoulders and hauled me in, explaining that the short stop was to change gears to slow the hoisting mechanism. I felt like a fish being hauled onto a pier, but was deeply grateful to be on a firm surface. They placed a headset on me, and the pilot asked me where we were going.

I was still pretty rattled, but managed to key up the mike. "Uh, to John Muir. It's that hospital over to your right about ten miles." I was secured in my seat next to the patient as the helicopter veered away from the mountain and headed off. Because of the speed of the Coast Guard aircraft, our flight time was only about three minutes, which gave me only enough time to start an IV and grab a blood pressure, no easy feat because my hands were still shaking badly. Our dispatch had called ahead to let John Muir know we were coming, and they knew that we were bringing a rock climber who had fallen. As we brought him into the trauma room and I gave report, I sank down in a chair and muttered to myself, "Never, never again."

Just when you thought you had it all figured out, this job found new and creative ways to embarrass you.

We had been asked to land at the scene of a shooting in Richmond and were given the cross streets of a park in the midst of a residential neighborhood. As we approached the area, the fire department called us on the radio.

"CALSTAR, you are directly overhead. We are in a park with no obstructions except some power lines to the north. The wind is negligible. The scene is secure." We looked down. Sure enough, there was a park, with two fire trucks nearby. This must be the place, I thought, though I was a bit puzzled by the structure across the street that was smoking; we had been called for a gunshot wound. Well, maybe he was a burn that got shot or something. The initial information we received was often wildly inaccurate, so this was nothing new.

There were bystanders milling about below, but the green expanse of lawn was clear. Well, OK. We were going to make a lot of wind, but these guys had worked with us a million times before, so they knew that. I was just hoping our downwash wouldn't stir up what appeared to be a still-smoldering fire below.

Carl, our pilot, spoke as we were circling the scene. His thoughts seemed to mirror mine. "I thought this was a gunshot wound. Oh well, nobody ever tells us anything. OK, I see the grassy area, and the wires on the north side. I don't see any other obstructions. Sure seems like an awful lot of people down there, though. After we land, get a few more firefighters or cops over here for aircraft security. Anybody see anything else?" We both murmured no, and Carl keyed up the mike to the ground. "Engine 52, this is CALSTAR. We have no obstructions. There seems to be a lot of people down there, so we'll need increased security. We're turning final."

"Copy that. We're ready for you," was the response. As we turned final, things started feeling very strange. The firefighters below were just standing there, staring at us, rather than hustling the crowd back. I looked for an ambulance, but saw none. Instead, there was a Red Cross disaster vehicle, the kind that hands out cookies and punch during a disaster. "That's funny," I thought. "I didn't know the Red Cross could do medical care unless there was a major disaster." My train of thought continued. "If the Red Cross is doing medical care, the medics must be really busy. But busy doing what?" The next thought came flooding in. "Oh, no. This must mean they're only doing first aid, with no advance life support. The patient probably isn't even packaged."

I was watching out the left window of the helicopter and saw a policeman trying to push a man in a wheelchair out of what was to be our LZ. We noticed bright yellow police tape everywhere. The fire department knew better than that—they knew we would blow that stuff away, and it could even get stuck in our rotor blades. It wouldn't hurt anything, but it would make a hell of a racket. We were just ten feet above the ground when Carl announced over the intercom, "You know, this just doesn't feel right. I'm aborting the landing. Too many people, and the LZ isn't secure." With that, he pulled up the collective and we veered off, back into the sky.

Just then, Engine 52 came back up on the radio. "Uh, CALSTAR, this is engine 52. We think you're at the wrong scene. We're a block north." Do you think you could have told us that before we nearly landed on some poor man in a wheel-chair?

We scooted up one block, and sure enough, there they were. After I got out of the helicopter, all the firefighters looked pretty sheepish. "Sorry about that," one of them said. "We thought you guys could read the street signs and knew this was where we wanted you."

Yeah. And we have X-ray vision, too.

Whether it's landing on the Bay Bridge or dangling precariously from a Coast Guard behemoth, flight nursing can certainly be dramatic and impressive to witness. That's why the CALSTAR helicopter was always a big attraction when we did demonstrations at community events. However, there were a few occasions when our attempts at high drama ended up closer to slapstick.

One was a fire awareness day in Contra Costa County. The residents of Orinda had gathered to see a display of the finest fire and EMS equipment their tax money could buy. The local fire department had brought out all its impressive apparatus: huge trucks, bright red and glistening in the sun. The entire battalion appeared in their uniforms, turnouts and helmets. The California Highway Patrol had brought its newest and shiniest vehicles, complete with all the latest gadgets. An ambulance crew was in attendance showing off their medical stuff, too. Clowns roamed the grounds, handing out balloons urging kids to just say no to drugs and gangs. A huge barbecue pit cranked out hot dogs and hamburgers. And at 1:30, CALSTAR was flying in to show off the state-of-the-art medical care available to the people in their time of need. They would all sleep soundly that night.

It was a sweltering day, and we were careful to keep hydrated. That day we had grabbed three Cokes as we ran out of quarters en route to the fair.

The crowd was standing anxiously, staring at the sky, as we popped over the ridge. The fire department had rigged an air-to-ground radio to the public address system, so everyone could hear our radio traffic. Firemen roamed the grounds checking their portable radios frequently as we approached. The landing zone had been carefully prepped ensuring no debris would be flung skyward with the winds generated as we landed. When we buzzed the LZ, reconning to ensure safety, mothers with small children headed into the building for safety. On short final, the noise and wind made created a dramatic backdrop heralding our arrival. Gently we settled onto the ground, all eyes on our grand spectacle.

After we shut down, the quiet was deafening. The doors on the helicopter opened simultaneously with a flourish. At that moment, three Coke cans rolled out and hit the ground with a decidedly undramatic tink, tink, tink. So much for instilling a sense of awe.

One of the more frightening community events for CALSTAR was the Boy Scout Jamboree. Every year the dreaded memo arrived, followed by frantic phone calls by the scheduled flight crew, who begged for somebody, anybody, to take the loathsome shift. Sometimes we could scam it off on the newbies, but they learned fast. Nobody volunteered two years in a row.

Why did everyone dread this particular event? Imagine, if you will, five hundred prepubescent boys, wired on Twinkies, rushing the helicopter. Their first target, invariably, was the antennas. We had a total of five external antennas mounted on the underside of the tailboom and belly, all of which were unbelievably expensive, fragile, and absolutely indispensable to the safe operation of the helicopter. One good grab and the antenna would snap off, leaving us out of service until it could be repaired. After they finished with the antennas, the Boy Scouts wanted in—in the helicopter, that is. They have some sort of internal radar that allows them to home in on, and then break, the most important and expensive equipment first.

On my last trip to the Boy Scout Jamboree, Carrie and I thought we had our bases covered. We had spoken with the troop leaders and laid down the rules: No running around the helicopter. No one inside the helicopter. We would post someone on either side of the tail rotor and one guard at each door to prevent small units from sneaking into the aircraft and causing havoc. Satisfied, we lifted off toward the fairground.

As we circled overhead, we were filled with a sense of foreboding. The ground below was teeming with kids, who looked like small ants swarming over the large field. They were everywhere. Tim regarded the landing zone with a sober eye. "Looks like a couple hundred of 'em. Soon as we get down, I want you to clear out. Take up your stations; I'll shut down as soon as possible. If they rush the helicopter, we'll have to clear out of there fast. Any questions?" We shook our heads, feeling as if we were landing in Vietnam.

When we began the landing, there was a brief bulge in the lines as the kids tried to surge forward. The Scout leaders, battling bravely, held them back. As soon as the skids hit the ground, Tim gave us a curt nod. "You're cleared out," he said grimly. We popped out, ready for combat, with our headsets still plugged in to the mothership.

The lines held, right up to the moment the rotors stopped turning. Despite the troop leaders' gallant efforts, the kids broke free. For a brief, horrible moment, I was frozen to the spot. Carrie, however, rose to the occasion. "Stop now!" she yelled. "I mean it! Nobody is coming any closer until everybody slows down." The kids slowed momentarily to a fast walk.

Two hours later, we realized we had lost. Kids continued to swarm over the helicopter like a plague of locusts. I had to do something. Anything. I tiptoed over to the telephone, dialed our group pager number and entered a nonsensical code. I then quickly ran back to the helicopter. "We've got a call!" I yelled. "Everybody back! Everybody back to the bleachers! Now! This may be a life or death situation!" Carrie and Tim looked at me as if I had finally gone over the edge. Then they looked at their pagers. "Why didn't they just call us on the portables?" Tim started to say, then finally caught on. "That's right! We must take off immediately! This is an actual real-life emergency call!" Sullenly, the Boy Scouts backed away. We lifted off in a cloud of dust, leaving our tormentors behind.

I'm told that CALSTAR still makes an annual appearance at the Boy Scout Jamboree. That's one part of the job I surely don't miss.

CHAPTER ELEVEN

Aren't You Afraid You're Going to Crash?

ONE of the first questions people ask flight nurses is, "Aren't you afraid you're going to crash in one of those helicopters?" The short answer is no. Statistically speaking, the most dangerous part of a twenty-four-hour shift at CALSTAR was the drive to and from work. I was more afraid crossing the San Mateo Bridge.

I should mention that I'm terrified of heights. To this day, I can't walk across the Golden Gate Bridge, and the glass elevators outside of skyscrapers make me sweat. Flying, however, has never bothered me.

Many people seem to have the idea that if something does go wrong in a helicopter, it means everyone plunges to their deaths, which is simply not true. Many in-flight emergencies, in fact, can be managed without danger to life or limb.

I always felt safe in the helicopter because the pilots' were exceptional, and I knew what they were comfortable with and what made them nervous. We were usually so in tune that we came to the same conclusions at the same time—an LZ wasn't safe, the weather was getting too lousy, and the like. Besides, the nurses were drilled over and over in emergency procedures, and we could run through the steps in our sleep.

We also placed a great deal of trust in the mechanics. Dave, our lead mechanic, took his job very seriously and would ground an aircraft immediately if there was a whiff of a problem. At times it was frustrating because we would miss flights, and therefore revenue, but the maintenance department was adamant about grounding the helicopter for even minor concerns.

CALSTAR also had a standing rule: If *any* one of us was uncomfortable with *any* aspect of a flight, we had the power to abort, no questions asked and without fear of recrimination. Generally, when we did abort a flight, it was after a simultaneous consensus. The trust was based on personal relationships; we operated as a family.

Pete, one of our senior pilots, was the safety officer for years. He was in charge of training, as well as developing, reviewing and revising emergency aviation policies. Once a year, for example, we would review the emergency water landing procedures. Pete would place Mae West flotation devices under our chairs, turn out the lights, then time us as we located them, got them on properly, simulated an exit from the aircraft, and inflated the vests.

The first couple of times we did this I was surprised. Despite having endured hundreds of those safety briefings that most people ignore on commercial jetliners, I learned that it takes a while to figure out how to get the thing out of the package, on and inflated, especially in the dark. That's why we needed to practice.

In a real emergency water landing, particularly at night, if we hadn't repeated this drill, we probably would have panicked and froze. But because of all the safety drills—which, frankly, get boring after a while—we would switch into an automatic mode whenever something went wrong.

One summer, Pete decided to start the drill for warning lights. The front panel of any helicopter has an array of lights that indicate various problems and their degree of severity. As we were flying along, he would simulate one or more of the warning lights and we would go through the required procedure. For the flight crew, most of the time it meant turning off the oxygen so as not to feed any flames, checking to see everything was secured, getting the appropriate radio call off to dispatch, and looking down to help locate an emergency landing zone.

One of the most serious was the warning light that indicated an engine was on fire. It became Pete's favorite drill. He would call out, "Fire warning light," and then turn the helicopter to the left and right while we looked out the window to see if we were trailing smoke. We'd turn off the O_2 and the pilot would shut down the indicated engine, leaving us flying on only one while we all looked for a safe place to land. He did this over and over again, and the repetition was getting to all of us.

At two o'clock one rainy morning, Andy, Pete, and I were activated to San Ramon for an auto rollover. Two a.m. is a special hour for us because it's when all the bars in California close, leaving the patrons staggering to their cars. This flight was no different. A young man who had been drinking had rolled his car on the freeway and was now trapped inside the vehicle. We trotted out to the helicopter, glad this was a quick scene call rather than an interfacility, which might have been hours long. As it was, we were overhead in less than five minutes. The CHP had shut down the freeway, and we landed uneventfully several hundred feet away. Since I was the primary nurse, I hefted the trauma bag onto my shoulder and hoofed it to the overturned car, which was surrounded by firefighters cutting it apart with the Jaws of Life. I could see a paramedic lying with half his body inside the vehicle, caring for the patient trapped inside.

The car was demolished, and pieces of it had fallen off as it had rolled down the road. Even without a report, I could tell he must have been traveling pretty fast to do that much damage.

A firefighter met me halfway. "Morning," he said amicably. "Got ourselves quite a mess. This is a twenty-one-year-old male who lost control of his car trying to outrun the cops. Story is he got caught at a sobriety checkpoint set up by the police, and when he realized where he was, he sped off. They got up to ninety miles an hour. He lost control about a half-mile up the road and rolled end over end to here. Right now he's dangling upside down in his seat belt, and we're trying to cut him out."

When we reached the vehicle, sure enough, I could see the paramedic trying to intubate him in that position. I knelt down in the broken glass and shouted in to the medic. "Is he breathing?"

"Not real well, and he's got a barely palpable pulse. I can see a head injury, but his facial bones are stable. He looks like he's got a flail chest on the left. You want to get in here and try a nasal tube? I can't get a good angle to see the vocal cords, so I don't think we're gonna get an oral one, and we won't be able to get him out for a while." I nodded and he crawled backward out of the wreck.

As I slid into the car on my back, over the glass and twisted metal, Andy trotted over and I explained the situation.

"OK," he said. "I'll give you the stuff as you go along." He opened the airway pouch and handed in the Neo Synephrine spray, which we hoped would prevent a nosebleed as I placed the tube. Then I held a high-flow oxygen mask over our patient's face while Andy pulled out the endotracheal tube and prepped it. The patient now had only agonal respirations. We had to hurry. If he stopped breathing altogether, it would be difficult, if not impossible, to thread the tube down the trachea.

Gently I pushed the tube into his nose. He didn't respond at all, another ominous sign. I waited for him to take a breath to advance it, but it didn't come. He had picked that moment to finally give up and try to die. I advanced the tube anyway and was rewarded with a fountain of partially digested food, which spattered over the front of my flight suit. I was clearly in the esophagus, and I was emptying his stomach through the tube. I pulled it back and tried again, with the same result. It was no use. I reached over and felt the carotid pulse—it was barely palpable at about ten.

"Andy, he's arrested. Hand me the cric kit." It was useless to try to do compressions with him dangling upside down, and I knew we had to get an airway before anything, so my plan was to perform a cricothyrotomy, a type of tracheostomy. I had done it on patients lying flat on a backboard, but never in the dark, in the rain, with a patient suspended upside down above me. There wasn't time to discuss the issue—our patient was nearly dead. To make matters worse, Andy wouldn't fit inside the vehicle with me, so he couldn't help. I was so scared my hands were shaking.

Andy handed me a Betadine swab to clean the neck. I palpated his throat and found what I hoped was the cricothyroid membrane. "OK, hand me the scalpel." He placed it in my hand, and I made an incision through the skin and between the rings of the trachea. There was very little bleeding, since our patient now had no blood pressure. As soon as I was through, I pushed my finger into the hole in the trachea so I wouldn't lose it, held my other hand out and asked for the trach hook. Andy handed it to me, and I put it in place to keep the surrounding tissue from falling into the incision. Then I sawed through the membrane to get to the trachea. "Trach tube," I said when I was done, and held my hand out again. Andy slapped the tube into my hand with the $ETCO_2$ detector already attached. I threaded it in, still holding the hook to keep back the skin. Once the trach tube eased into place, I inflated the balloon to achieve a seal.

"I think I got it," I said as I began bagging him. We had an airway. I secured the tube by wrapping a cloth tape around his neck and tying it.

"Andy, he's still got no blood pressure. We have to get him out of here now." The firefighters, who had held up till the cric was completed, resumed their efforts. Since the paramedics had been able to start an IV before our arrival, they got busy pushing the emergency medications. The firefighters handed me a blanket to protect myself from the sparks and glass as they worked, and under the blanket I continued to bag the patient while lying on my back in the damp darkness with him dangling above me.

After what seemed to be an eternity, they finally got the car pulled apart, and I held our patient's neck in alignment as we eased him onto the backboard. Now that he was getting oxygen and emergency medications, he had a faint pulse again. As fast as we could, we finished packaging him and loaded him on the helicopter for the seven-minute flight to John Muir.

En route we found he did have a blood pressure, but not much of one. Andy started a second large-bore IV and we poured in the fluids. We barely had enough time to radio a report to the hospital to let them know what we were bringing. We did a hot offload and rolled into the trauma room at a full run. As we moved him over to the gurney, he arrested again. Andy and I backed out of the room as the trauma team took over.

We retired to the back room to start our never-ending paperwork, but I couldn't concentrate; there was still too much adrenaline. Putting in that cric was one of the most frightening experiences of my life. Andy put his arms around me. "You did great," he said. I took several deep breaths, and slowly my heart rate came back down to normal.

On the flight home, Andy and I were trying to get our paperwork done so we could get to bed. It had been a long day, and that flight drained what was left of my energy. Suddenly Pete called out, "Fire warning light." Andy and I groaned, put the paperwork down, and went through the drill.

"OK, oxygen is off," Andy recited tiredly. "I'm getting off a call to dispatch. I'm looking—no smoke or flames on either side."

"Very good," Pete said.

"Do ya have to do that every night, Pete?" I whined as we flew on through the night.

"Come on, Janice, you know that the best time to do drills is at night when everybody's tired. Stop bitching." I sighed, reaching again for the paperwork. He was right, but I wasn't in the mood for a lecture.

Two hours later, at 4:30 a.m., we were just finishing up restocking and charting when we called John Muir. Our patient had died twenty minutes after arrival.

The adrenaline was now long gone, replaced by an overwhelming weariness. "Andy, I gotta get into bed. I'm exhausted." I went into the bedroom, pulled off my stinking flight suit and fell into bed. I was asleep almost instantly.

After what seemed like only a few minutes, the phone rang. I reached over, knocking it onto the floor as I answered it with a mumble. I glanced at the clock. It was 6:15 a.m.

"You're going to Delta Memorial for a gunshot wound," said Elise, our dispatcher. "Sorry to get you out of bed again. You're taking him to John Muir."

Andy stirred on the other side of the room. "We got a flight?" he asked, groping for his flight suit. I nodded as Elise gave me the information. Andy jumped up and pounded on the wall. "Pete, we got a flight!" he yelled as he zipped up his flight suit and scanned the ground for his boots.

We had been activated to a small hospital in the Delta to transport a thirty-five-year-old patient who had been dumped outside their ER twenty minutes ago. He had been shot and was in bad shape. We trudged out to the helicopter in the lightening morning sky. This was our fifth flight of the shift, and I was exhausted. Thankfully, it was a relatively short distance to Delta Memorial, and our flight to John Muir would be short, too. We landed in the parking lot, where an ambulance met us.

We walked into the ER to find an enormous man, intubated, lying on a gurney and surrounded by feverish activity. The doctor was placing a chest tube as we came in.

"Boy, are we glad to see you," he said. "The staff found this guy about half an hour ago lying in the ER parking lot. Somebody must have dumped him there. He has four gunshot wounds—two in his right chest, and two in his umbilical area. No idea when he was shot, or with what, or what range. The chest X-ray showed a pneumothorax on the right. He's real hypotensive, and we have two big IVs. We've ordered some O-negative blood, 'cause we didn't have time to cross-match him. It should be here in a minute. His blood pressure is only eighty, and we've been pouring fluids in him. I called the trauma doc over at John Muir and they're waiting for you."

Andy and I went to work getting him ready. A nurse pushed the copied chart and X-rays into my hand, and another brought us two units of blood, one of which we hung right away. As quickly as we could, we packaged him up and, with the help of six people, managed to move him over to our litter. He was so big we had a hard time getting the belts around him. We pushed him out to the waiting ambulance for the short ride back to where Pete was waiting.

When we arrived at the helicopter, I slid out and loaded in our bags, the X-rays, chart and blood. I turned on the oxygen, then trotted back to the ambulance where Andy was waiting with the patient. "OK, ready for you." We pulled the patient out of the back of the ambulance and rolled him over to the helicopter.

As we pulled him up, Pete held up his hand. "Oh, shit. How much does this guy weigh?" he asked, pulling out his flight calculator. My heart sank. We hadn't thought to check weight and balance, and since it had been only a short ride to Delta, our gas tank was almost full, adding a significant amount of weight to the helicopter.

I looked at the man and rummaged through the chart quickly. "They have him down as about 280 pounds—around 125 kilos."

Pete punched the numbers into the computer, shaking his head. "I'm sorry, no way is that going to work. We'd be way over on weight. If I'd have known, I could have flown around burning off some fuel while you guys were inside. I'm really sorry." Andy and I looked at one another, trying to decide what to do.

"Put him back in the ambulance," Andy said to the paramedics. "Sorry to do this to you, but we're hijacking you. You've got to take us by ground." Normally the drive to John Muir from Delta would be around twenty minutes, but we were now facing morning rush-hour traffic. Still, Andy was right; we had no other option.

Andy turned back to Pete. "Call dispatch and let them know—and tell them to contact John Muir and give them an updated ETA. We'll call report to them directly from the radio in the ambulance. You can fly over there and meet us. It'll probably take about half an hour." Pete nodded and we jumped back into the ambulance, setting off with lights and siren.

All the way to the trauma center, we frantically pushed fluids. I kept kicking myself—I should have known to ask for the weight as soon as we got there and relayed the information to Pete. As the secondary nurse, that was part of my job. Andy had the grace not to mention my oversight. We worked silently as the ambulance wound its way through bumper-to-bumper traffic. I looked shakily at my watch. It was 7:30, and the new crew should be in quarters by the time we got home.

After an eternity we pulled into John Muir's ER. Remarkably, our patient had not deteriorated en route, but he remained a very sick man. We gave report, knocked out a quick chart, and headed back for the helipad where Pete had flown in to meet us.

The flight back to quarters was quiet as Andy and I again tried to finish up the chart. The new crew was waiting for us, and we had radioed ahead to let them know they needed to restock the bags. My exhaustion was now complete, and I decided to try and sleep an hour or two at quarters before I went home, since I didn't think it was safe to do the forty-five-minute drive. I looked out the window and saw we were just about back at the airport.

Then Pete keyed up the intercom. "Fire warning light."

I had had enough. Five flights, up all night, a middle-of-the-night cric, and then the stupid oversight that meant we had to take a patient by ground. "Fuck you, Pete. Not now," I said, not even looking up at the warning panel.

"I'm not fooling," Pete answered sternly. "We got a fire warning light."

I looked up and, sure enough, we really did have a light. We launched into that automatic mode: Pete pulled the throttle all the way back to shut down the engine, then banked to the right and left as Andy and I craned our necks to look for smoke or flames. I reached around and ensured the oxygen was shut off. There was no time to call dispatch.

We were about thirty feet off the ground when Pete came up on the intercom. "We're doing a run-on landing, so make sure you're all secure. This could be bumpy." With that, he flared the helicopter slightly to decrease our forward speed, then pushed the nose down. We hit the runway and skidded for a good forty feet, coming to a stop with a lurch. The rotors flung forward, then back again. Pete pulled the throttle back to shut down the remaining engine. Only two minutes had elapsed since he called the light.

Beth, Harry, and Tim, the oncoming crew, had watched the landing from quarters and now came running out toward us as I unsteadily climbed out of the helicopter. There was no fire. I stood dumbly looking at the engine cowlings, expecting them to erupt into flames at any moment. Beth ran up to me yelling, "Are you guys all right? What happened?"

The night had taken its toll, and I burst into tears. "We had a fire warning light and the patient was too fat and we had to go in traffic and he was shot and the guy was hanging upside down and I had to do a cric...." She put her arms around me as I babbled. Andy climbed out, gray and shaking, too, but at least coherent.

"We just had a fire warning light that we thought was real," he said, stepping down from the skid. "That's why we did the run-on landing. We've had a pretty hellish shift. I'll tell you all about it later. We got to get Dave out here to check the helicopter." Beth gently propelled me, still sniveling, into quarters.

"Janice, how about a cup of tea, OK?" I nodded, trying to stop the tears. She sat me down and handed me some hot tea. Andy followed us in, sat heavily on the couch, and swore under his breath.

The next day we got everything sorted out. The fire warning light had been caused by a broken wire, and we were never in any danger. Our large patient did fine once he got to the OR to get his holes fixed. I went home and slept like a dead woman.

That fire warning light haunted me for the rest of my tenure, although we never had to do another run-on landing. We did, however, have a run in with another potential menace. We told this story any time a visitor noticed the duck decals—two and a half ducks to be precise—on the pilot's door of the helicopter.

Beth and I had just returned from a butt-numbing, four-hour flight with a cardiac patient from Visalia to San Francisco. "They certainly didn't design those seats with comfort in mind, did they?" she said as we ambled into quarters, clutching the patient's five-page chart. As we got into the office, I picked up the phone to call dispatch to get the flight number for the log. James, our dispatcher that day, answered.

"Hey, James, it's Janice. You got a flight number for me?"

"Sure. It's 10136C497F. And you missed a flight while you were gone, too," he said.

"Rats. What was it?"

"A shark attack in Santa Cruz. Heard the guy almost had his leg chewed off. Lifeflight handled it."

"We miss all the good stuff. A shark attack would have been a lot more fun than a cardiac patient."

"Sure would have been. There's a lot of media over this one, so check out the news tonight."

"OK. Thanks. You can show us as back in service now."

Later that night we watched the news and sure enough, there was Lifeflight, our competitor in the air ambulance business, in one of the lead stories. Apparently the patient had been surfing when the shark grabbed him by the leg, shook him violently, then let go. This is characteristic of shark attacks—they usually strike once, injuring the prey, then come in for a second, usually lethal bite. Sharks often mistake surfers for their favorite food, because a person with his arms and legs dangling over a surfboard appears from below to be a sea lion. Often they make only the initial attack and then swim off. This guy had the presence of mind to pound the shark on his nose, which also may have helped save his life. In any case, the shark didn't come back, and he managed to paddle to shore, bleeding heavily from a deep laceration in his thigh, which had partially severed the femoral artery.

Shark attacks are relatively rare in northern California, and they usually garnered a lot of media attention. "That would have been our flight," Beth said, shaking her head as we watched the news story. "Damn, they've probably already got another decal stuck on."

There were several minutes of footage of the Lifeflight crew landing on the beach, assessing the patient, then taking off again. It was great coverage, and we were, quite frankly, jealous. Over the years we had established a friendly rivalry with the competing EMS helicopters in northern California, but particularly with Lifeflight, since we shared the same response zone. (We called them Lifefright, and they called us Deathstar.) They had got the last two shark attacks, both of which would have been our calls if we hadn't been busy. Like World War II flying aces who kept track of their kills with swastikas painted on the sides of their airplanes, Lifeflight already had two small sharks proudly decorating their helicopter. We all felt it was high time CALSTAR had one, too. "Next one, Beth," I said. "We'll get the next one. We'll get that shark decal yet."

Several years passed with no shark attacks. Late one night, Carrie, Carl and I were activated to Richmond for an assault. It was three o'clock in the morning, and I was less than pleased to be dragged out of my warm bed. The mid-December night was moonless, with a few wisps of fog in some of the deeper valleys. We had made the same flight hundreds of times before. Dispatch instructed us to rendezvous with the paramedics at Brookside's helipad. Eleven minutes later, Carl gently settled us onto the ground.

I grabbed the trauma bag and walked quickly over to the waiting ambulance. As I opened the doors, I was engulfed by an overpowering odor of alcohol. "Jeez," I said to the medic as I climbed in, "how much has this guy been drinking?"

"A lot," he answered, taping the IV in place. "This is Mr. Jones. He was found unconscious on a street corner about half an hour ago." He pointed to our patient's face, which was covered with abrasions. He also had two black eyes, one of which was swollen shut. "We're guessing he was assaulted, but we don't know with what, and he doesn't remember the event. He started waking up after the fire department got there. His skull is stable and the rest of his exam is negative, except for the heavy odor of alcohol. He claims he has no past medical problems and denies taking any medication, but his level of consciousness markedly improved after we gave him some Narcan to reverse any opiates. But he's still not oriented to person, place and time, so we figured he should go to the trauma center to make sure he isn't altered because of the head injury." I listened carefully as he spoke, and started my own primary exam.

Part of a neurological exam is to ensure the patient is alert and oriented times four: person, place, time, and purpose. If he can't come up with all those answers, we regard him as having an altered level of consciousness and have to seek the reason. Alcohol obscures the brain's sensorium, and we cannot be sure that the altered level is not due to head injury rather than alcohol alone. To worsen the odds, the liver is where the body makes the clotting factors that keep us from bleeding to death. Liver function is damaged by chronic alcoholism, and these patients are more prone to intercranial bleeds after relatively minor head trauma. In this case, the gentleman clearly had some facial trauma, but we had no way of knowing if he was just drunk or had some serious pathology going.

Mr. Jones was lying on the gurney in full spinal precautions, watching me with his one good eye. "Mr. Jones," I said, "I'm Janice, one of the nurses on the helicopter. What happened to you tonight?"

"Don't know," he replied, slurring his words. "I was just sittin' there, and they came and got me."

"Where do you hurt?"

"Don't hurt, don't hurt at all," he answered, despite the obvious injuries. That made sense. He was well anesthetized with alcohol and God only knows what else.

"How much have you had to drink tonight?" I asked.

"Oh, 'bout two beers," Mr. Jones slurred, and smiled at me, revealing a dentist's nightmare. He was missing quite a few teeth, and the remaining ones were clearly rotting through. I glanced at the medic who rolled his eyes. Every drunk in the world always answers that question the same way: "Oh, two beers," even when faced with the overwhelming evidence that they must have consumed at least ten times that much alcohol.

"I see," I said. "Have you taken anything else? Recreational drugs?"

"Nope. Don't do that shit." As he was talking, I took his left arm to inspect his antecubital veins. Most people are right-handed, so the left antecubital is the first choice for illicit IV drug use. Again, Mr. Jones wasn't exactly being honest. His veins were obviously well used, and there appeared to be some fresh track marks.

"If you say so," I said, knowing it was useless to point out the inconsistencies in his story. "We're going to take you over to John Muir to have them check you out, OK? And we want you to stay still in case your neck has been injured."

"All right," he answered, and promptly dozed off. We loaded our friend into the helicopter and lifted off into the dark night. Occasionally he would wake up, mumble to himself, wiggle around, then fall back to sleep. Carrie and I were both rather unimpressed, and she promptly began to fill in the chart as soon as we had safely cleared the helipad. I set about hooking up the monitors and trying to keep Mr. Jones still. As I expected, all his vital signs were stable, and his oxygenation was perfect on room air. Still, just to cover the bases, I put on a nasal cannula with a couple liters of oxygen.

To fly to John Muir, we had to go over a small range of hills that separates the bay from the Mount Diablo Valley, where the trauma center for Contra Costa County is located. It's mostly parkland or protected open space, and at night from the air there is a dark band separating the valley, with no lights to use as reference points.

Suddenly, we heard a loud thud and the helicopter snapped violently to the right. Instantly, both Carrie and I were at attention and beginning emergency procedures. "Everybody hang on," Carl said, as he carefully tested the flight controls. Already I was looking down at the ground, trying to make out a safe landing zone in case the engines shut down and we went into autorotation. (Helicopters, like airplanes, can glide to a controlled landing when they lose engines, since the descent will keep the rotors turning and provide some lift.

But we would need a flat, safe LZ very close by.) Of course, being an absolutely black night, we could see nothing. Besides, we all knew there were precious few flat spots until we got past the ridge line.

Carl quickly keyed up the mike. "Everything is working, I have control of the helicopter. I have no warning lights. There's no place to land out here, so I'm going to continue to John Muir for now. Keep looking for landing zones as we proceed. Get a call off to dispatch. And please turn off the oxygen."

At that point, none of us had any idea what that thud might have been. We all listened intently. Even though the nurses are not pilots, after years of flying we became accustomed to the normal noises of each particular aircraft and could tell immediately if something was wrong. I could hear nothing unusual, and we seemed to be flying normally.

John Muir was now only about three minutes away. If we continued as we were, we could reach the hospital helipad, as long as nothing failed. I held my breath and my heart was pounding as we got closer and closer. Mr. Jones, seemingly unaware of the incident, continued to mumble and wriggle himself out of the straps that held him to the backboard. We all scanned for any unusual change in pitch or vibration. Finally, after what seemed like hours, Carl safely settled us down on the helipad.

Carrie immediately got on the radio. "CALSTAR base, CALSTAR One. We are down at John Muir at 3:32. Show us as being out of service due to an unusual occurrence. Will landline when able." Meanwhile, I watched Carl closely and as soon as the skids were on the ground he nodded his head, and I leaped out of the helicopter to survey any damage. My headset was still plugged in, and I was ready to quickly get away from the aircraft if any parts appeared to be falling or flying off.

What I saw was not what I was expecting. Hanging limply out of one of the jet engines was the head of a mallard duck, with the rest of his body inside the intake. The side of the helicopter was smeared with blood and duck guts. I was so shocked it took me a minute to react.

"Uh, Carl," I said over the intercom while the engines were still running, "I think I see what the problem is."

"What is it?" he asked anxiously. "Are the engine cowlings intact?"

"Yup. There's a duck hanging out of one of the engines. Or at least part of a duck."

"What? What did you say?"

"A duck. God rest his poor little duck soul. He's in a better place now." Despite, or perhaps because of our terror during the past five minutes, I had to laugh.

Carl shut down, and we offloaded Mr. Jones as he continued to mutter to himself. We gave a brief report to the trauma team and headed for the back room to write up the chart. Both Carrie and I were shaking and we sat down to take several deep breaths. Carrie then picked up the phone to call dispatch and get Phyllis, our mechanic, to come and survey the damage. It was now four in the morning.

As soon as we could pull the chart together, Carrie and I ran back out to the helipad. We found Carl peering into the engine intake with a flashlight. He had removed the engine cowlings and small bits of duck were scattered over the ground. "I don't see anything seriously damaged, but there's blood and feathers all over the engine deck," he said, climbing down. "This helicopter isn't going anywhere for a while. You guys should call a cab to get back to base. I'll stay till Phyllis gets here." He picked up a plastic bag, and heaved it into the garbage bin next to the helipad.

"What was that?" I asked.

"The remains of Mr. Duck."

"You can't just throw him in the garbage," I objected. "We have to go bury him or something. Say a few words."

"Janice," Carl said, getting irritated with my kidding, "you don't seem to understand. That duck could have killed us."

Carl was right. Bird strikes are a serious threat in aviation. There have been cases where a bird has struck the windshield, coming through and killing the pilot. Birds have also been sucked into jet intakes, shutting down engines, usually at the most critical time of takeoff. If we had hit the bird a little lower, or if it had come through the Plexiglas, we could have been toast. This time it was the duck's turn.

Several days later, I went out to preflight while Phyllis was there doing the daily inspection. I noticed some new decals on the pilot's door. I inspected them curiously as Phyllis came off the ladder, wiping her greasy hands on a rag.

"We were lucky," she said. "We didn't have any major damage from the bird strike. You guys must have flown right into a flock of them. Don't ask me what a flock of ducks was doing at a thousand feet at three o'clock in the morning."

"A flock of them?" I asked.

"Yeah. When we put all the parts together, we found two and a half ducks. So you finally got your decals—two and a half ducks. Lifeflight, eat your heart out."

CHAPTER TWELVE

The Day Oakland Burned

"LADIES and gentlemen, we will be landing at San Francisco International Airport in just a few minutes. Kindly pass any glasses to the aisle for collection, and return your seats and tables to their original positions."

I closed my eyes and said a silent prayer of thanks. The AAMES (Association of Air Medical Emergency Services) conference had been the hardest four days I had endured in years. I felt my abdomen, expecting to find my liver edging close to my navel. If I never saw another bottle of tequila again, it would be too soon. I desperately wanted to get home, hug Mark and Roscoe, take a long shower, and sleep in my own bed.

Rose, who was sitting on the other side of the aisle, woke up and started gathering her luggage. She leaned over to me. "This has been quite the field trip, huh? Hey, we're working together the day after tomorrow. Think you'll be recovered by then?"

"Doubt it," I answered. "I'm sick of looking at you." We grinned at each other and she squeezed my hand.

I glanced over at Andy, who was rummaging through his bag. Like mine, it was overflowing with T-shirts and cheap souvenirs we had picked up at the conference. "Hey, Janice, do you know what I did with my beeper?" he asked. "I can't find it."

"I have it, remember? I took it away from you on the way to Tampa. Guess you can have it back now." I pawed through my own bag and pulled out a smelly shirt I had been wearing the previous night. It was heavy with more than 150 pins, which I had collected from various flight programs around the country.

"Janice, you are such a pin slut," Andy said, shaking his head.

"I worked hard for those pins," I responded. "Oh, here's your beeper. It's official. The party's over. We're going to have to pretend we're adults again."

We landed and disembarked. As we were trudging through the baggage claim, Andy's beeper went off. "I can't believe this," he muttered. "We haven't been on the ground more than fifteen minutes. Would you guys get my bag for me? I'll meet you at the carousel." He headed off for a bank of phones.

Rose looked over at me and smiled. "Welcome home."

The 1992 AAMES conference was in Tampa, and I was up before dawn to get ready for the flight. As I grabbed my bag and headed for the door, I realized I had forgotten to kiss Mark goodbye. I made a quick about face and ran into the bedroom, where he was still wrapped in the gentle arms of sleep. I leaned over and whispered in his ear, "Bye, honey. I'm off to AAMES. I'll call you with the hotel's phone number when I get there. My flight information is on the dining room table. Love you."

Mark curled himself deeper into the covers. "Don't drink too much," he mumbled. "And bring me back lots of loot, OK?"

I scooped up Roscoe and gave him a quick kiss. "You two bachelors behave yourselves while I'm gone."

Attending AAMES is a rite of passage—you're not truly a flight nurse until you've been initiated by spending a full week too hung over to sit up. Now the conferences have become marginally respectable, but in the early days of helicopter medicine, they were really nothing more than drinkfests. This was my third one, and I'd be attending with Andy and Rose. It didn't take us long to get into the spirit—we began in the air with a breakfast of complimentary Bloody Marys. "You know, we're already in trouble," I said. "God help us."

We arrived at Tampa International Airport at the same time as a contingent from Pennsylvania, a group of hard-partying flight nurses we knew well. There was much squealing, chattering and hugging as we caught up. All of us would be staying at a cut-rate hotel across the street from the Hyatt, the official lodgings for the conference. We had found in previous years that a cheap hotel's management was more tolerant of our late-night activities than the more respectable chains. We piled into three taxis, seven bodies in each, and headed for the city.

Forty-five minutes later, we were in the lobby of the Surf Hotel. As we approached the desk, the manager, who had been quietly reading the paper, looked up with alarm. He regarded us suspiciously as we checked in. Frank, one of the Pennsylvania nurses, popped open a beer from his portable cooler.

"What convention are you with?" he asked. "Hey, you over there. No open containers in the lobby. Yeah, I'm talking to you. You can buy booze in the bar, but ya can't bring your own in here."

Andy, always the diplomat, tried to take control of the situation. "Glad to meet you, sir. I'm the chief flight nurse at California Shock/Trauma Air Rescue. We're with the aeromedical conference." He turned to Frank. "Now, Frank, you know better than that. The gentleman's right. Put that away. We want to make a good impression, don't we?" He turned back to the manager and unleashed a dazzling smile. "Don't worry, we're professionals."

Soon after, we were pulling chairs around the pool and Andy headed to the bar for the first round. "Hey!" a voice yelled from the other side of the pool. "Andy! Janice! Rose! Over here!" It was George and Skip, two flight nurses from a program in North Carolina called MAMA, an acronym for their sponsoring hospital. Their exploits at AAMES were legendary, and we affectionately referred to them as the MAMA's Boys. As we pulled up our towels and prepared to join them, the Pennsylvanians started to file in. Frank was grinning and hauling a fifth of tequila. I knew it was over.

The rest of the evening was more or less a fog. I vaguely remember all of us being thrown out of the pool at 2:00 a.m. and trying to sneak into the Hyatt's hot tub around three. Another group of flight nurses from North Dakota joined us in our hotel room around four, along with a cold case of beer. The next thing I remember was the shrill buzz of the alarm clock at 7:00 a.m.

I looked around the room. Rosie was lying on the other bed, fully dressed but looking rather wrinkled. Andy lay on the floor, snoring and curled up in my bedspread. The MAMA's Boys were lying in a heap of wet towels. Rose opened her eyes and stared blearily at me. "God, what a night," she whispered. "Am I still alive?"

"I don't know about you," I said, "but I wish I was dead." I stumbled over Andy as I headed for the showers. "Oops, sorry. Make way, coming through." Andy sat up carefully, holding his head.

"Whose shorts are these?" he asked, looking down at the soggy swim trunks he was wearing.

"They're Skip's. You didn't have any trunks to wear in the hot tub last night, so he gave you his. You should appreciate that—he was wearing them at the time."

I leaned against the shower wall, praying the hot water would wash away the toxins. There was a class at eight that morning that had us all thrilled—at least it had sounded thrilling the day before. A famous professor of anatomy was scheduled to dissect a cadaver in one of the huge meeting rooms. As a freshman studying anatomy in college, I had studiously avoided even looking at cadavers because of squeamishness. Obviously I had gotten over this hurdle, and I was eager to get a review of the actual structures we so frequently dealt with in the field.

Now it seemed like a really bad idea. I could barely stand up, my stomach was in utter turmoil, and my head felt like it would explode with each heartbeat. I wasn't even sure I could walk to the convention center, let alone watch a postmortem dissection. "Please, somebody just shoot me now," I whispered to myself, closing my eyes and letting the water wash over my face.

After a breakfast of hot tea and dry toast, we trudged over to the lecture through rush-hour congestion. The exhaust fumes were overwhelming, and the jackhammers from a nearby construction site drilled into my skull. Despite a large-brimmed hat and dark glasses, I cringed at the bright sunlight.

The convention center was a cavernous affair divided into

many large lecture halls. We milled around aimlessly, unsure of where the class was to be held. Then we caught a whiff of what could only be cadaver. There is a unique odor associated with the anatomy lab—formaldehyde mixed with the smell of a dead body—that defies description. Once that smell has registered, it is locked forever into the memory banks. There is no smell quite as repulsive in this world.

"You know," Rose said as we found the doorway, "maybe we shouldn't hog all the good seats in front." Andy and I nodded as we sidled into the room, trying not to look at the dissection table.

We sat down just as the professor strode into the room, resplendent in his flowing white lab coat. "Good morning!" he boomed into the microphone, causing several of my cohorts to clutch their foreheads. The professor continued, unaware of the pain he was inflicting. "It is a pleasure to be teaching such an accomplished group of medical professionals. I realize many of you have not returned to the anatomy lab since your initial training. I hope today's lecture will be informative and stimulating." As he spoke, he whipped off the plastic that covered the body. Television monitors revealed a close-up view of the wizened cadaver's face and neck, with its mouth slightly ajar. We all recoiled in horror. Not one of our group was prepared to witness such a sight.

The professor continued, oblivious to our reaction. "Today, we will start with the dissection of the neck and trachea, as the emergency management of the airway is a top priority for this group." He made a large incision and began to busily saw away, and soon he had removed a large section of the trachea, including the larynx. He raised it up as if it were a trophy. Then he held the larynx to the camera as he reviewed the various structures. Giant vocal cords loomed in the monitors.

My stomach was churning, but I tried to concentrate. If I had gone through the trouble of getting here, I thought, I might as well learn something. The professor continued to deftly fillet the neck, describing structures as he cut. I turned to Rose, who was intently studying her shoes. "Rosie, are you OK?" I whispered.

"Just fine," she whispered back, still staring at the ground.

Our lecturer, now having completely macerated the neck, turned his attention to the chest. Brandishing a sternal saw, he applied it to the thorax with great enthusiasm. This was followed by a gleeful attack on the rib cage with huge rib cutters. The noises from the front sounded as if he were squashing bullfrogs, and I felt my head starting to swim. Andy had beads of sweat on his face while Rosie continued to stare steadily at the floor.

But the good doctor was not yet done. He proceeded to identify and rip out all the major structures in the thorax, explaining the various body parts in detail. The television camera was now trained on an empty chest cavity, and unmentionable fluids dripped down the inner wall. I was sure I couldn't stand much more.

After the discussion of the thorax was complete, our professor paused, building dramatic tension. "And now," he boomed, "I would like to present you with the most fascinating aspect of human anatomy." Again he paused as he grappled with the skull. "I present you with...the human brain." With a flourish he pulled out the glistening, dripping gray mass by the brainstem and held it aloft.

I felt the room spin and I lunged for an exit. I couldn't breathe. My stomach was in my throat, and I needed to find a bathroom in a hurry. It was all I could do to stagger down the hall. Thankfully, there was a bathroom next door, and I crawled into a booth, retching. On either side, I could hear other occupants performing the same task. I sank to the floor, mortified. How could a simple dissection have such devastating effects? After all, we saw a lot worse than that in our daily work.

I couldn't face my colleagues and, after getting cleaned up, I decided to return to the hotel room and crawl back into bed. I slipped out the door, hoping no one would see me.

To my surprise, our entourage was milling around in the lobby when I got back to the hotel. Suddenly Frank appeared, yelling, "Hey, they're giving away free beer out here!" Someone dragged me out and put a bottle in my hand. I glanced at it and realized to struggle was useless. I took a tentative sip.

And thus began another day at AAMES.

Now we were back in San Francisco, and the sound of Andy's beeper had hauled us into reality. Andy returned from the phones with a dark scowl on his face. "What's wrong?" I asked. "Is everything OK at home?"

"Oh, home is fine. But CALSTAR isn't. While we've been off pickling ourselves, all hell has broken loose. Carrie's father-in-law had emergency surgery, and she had to go home to help. That left the helicopter with only a skeleton crew, and everybody's been working thirty-six-hour shifts to keep it covered. Now Mike's sick, and there's nobody to work tomorrow." Nobody except us. There was only one possible solution: Rose would work a thirty-six-hour shift starting that night, and I would work a thirty-six starting the next morning. Of course, Mark would be less than thrilled to have me away for another day and a half, but that was the only way to keep the helicopter in service.

The next morning, I got to work as Rosie was getting out

of bed. "Did you guys fly last night?" I asked as I dumped my groceries on the counter.

"Thank heavens, no," Rosie said as she reached for the coffee pot. "Didn't turn a rotor. First decent night's sleep I've had for a week. Thank you, beeper gods." We headed down to the helicopter for the morning's preflight.

It was a beautiful, warm October day with clear skies, and by the time we were done with our morning duties, it was close to eighty degrees with a brisk wind from the south. California had been in the midst of a four-year drought, which turned the hills a deep golden color from the drying vegetation.

By lunchtime we were in quarters watching the news as we ate. There was a minor story about a small brush fire in the Oakland Hills, an area of swanky homes overlooking the East Bay and connected by narrow, winding roads. Tim watched the screen intently. "God help those guys if they ever get a real fire going up there," he said. "They'd never get it out. Those fire trucks would never get up those tiny roads, and with this drought the whole state is one large tinderbox. Everything would explode."

Mid-afternoon we were dispatched to Briones Reservoir Park for a mountain bike accident—a possible broken back. Briones Reservoir is one ridge past the Oakland Hills, and as we approached we noticed a small plume of smoke rising from Grizzly Peak. I contacted the fire department, who reassured us that a crew was already on its way. The small brush fire had reignited, but all was under control. Satisfied that things were in hand, we turned our attention to the landing zone.

We spotted the firefighter at the exact coordinates we had been given, and Tim made a few lazy circles before we landed on the open ridge top. I walked over to the firefighter and dropped the trauma bag heavily at my feet.

"Your patient should be here in a few minutes," he said. "The medics were just finishing packaging him, and then they'll bring him up here. He's doing OK—moving all four— but he looks like he's in a lot of pain."

"We timed this well, then. Hey, have you seen the smoke from Grizzly Peak in Oakland?" I pointed to the wisp we had noticed on the way in.

"Yeah," he answered, "I feel sorry for the guys in Oakland Fire. Must be ninety degrees out there by now. Won't be much fun putting that thing out. But, thankfully, it's not in our jurisdiction. We'll call them tonight after dinner and see how things went."

As we spoke, the ambulance came up the hill, groaning over every rut in the road. I could imagine that this short ride must be intensely painful for the patient as they bounced along the firebreak. Rose had come over to meet me, and together we loaded him into the aircraft for the eight-minute ride to the hospital. He was stable, but we needed a lot of morphine to keep him comfortable.

When we returned to the helicopter after dropping the patient at John Muir, we were stopped cold by the sight that met us as we walked out the ambulance doors. To the west, over the top of Grizzly Peak, a huge angry cloud of black smoke rose almost two thousand feet in the air. We stood and stared, dumbfounded, at the huge mushroom cloud. Tim wandered out from the cafeteria, carrying his ever-present cup of coffee. "Looks like that thing means business this time," he observed.

We didn't have a chance to respond because our pagers went off. We sprinted to the helicopter and cranked up the radios before starting the engines. "CALSTAR Base, CALSTAR One. Copy activation. Do you have further?"

"CALSTAR One, you have been activated to Grizzly Peak for an injured firefighter. Alameda County is declaring a level two disaster, and there are multiple agencies statewide responding, including CDF air ops. There are multiple aircraft in the area, and air ops are being coordinated by CDF on local frequency. We have been advised to have pilot contact CDF air ops prior to approaching area."

"Copy for CALSTAR One. We have an ETA of eight minutes to scene. Will advise when we get airborne. Please contact both John Muir and Brookside for burns and check their availability."

As we lifted off, the huge cloud of smoke appeared to be getting larger. We could clearly see walls of flame, hundreds of feet high, engulfing the hills. Trees dried by years of drought, especially eucalyptus, were exploding. We could see several helicopters circling the fire and dropping water from Bambi Buckets. These collapsible canvas buckets are suspended below the helicopter, and they're filled by being dropped into a lake or pool. Once the pilot is over the fire, the bucket opens and releases the water.

For a few minutes, we were all speechless. "My Lord," I breathed, "how can they possibly put this thing out?" A hot dry wind was whipping up, pushing the flames eastward toward the exclusive communities of Orinda and Moraga.

Rose dialed up Alco to receive instructions for our landing zone. The channel was flooded with traffic from all the ambulances, and we could hear requests to call in aid from around the state. We were beginning to understand the enormity of this fire and the potentially devastating impact it might have.

Seeing Alco was too busy to talk, Rose switched to the countywide fire frequency, which was just as jammed. We could hear the frantic calls of the firefighters requesting help. Some of them were withdrawing due to the intensity of the heat and flames that were rapidly spreading out of control. We heard the frustration and fear in their voices as everyone realized this was no longer a simple blaze. It was about to graduate to a firestorm.

Seven or eight helicopters flew over the area with buckets, and several fixed-wing air tankers were higher overhead. The smoke was obscuring a good deal of the sky by that point, and the aircraft were darting in and out of the active fire area, which now spread out over many square miles.

Tim turned us away from the fire and circled Briones Reservoir till the CDF's air incident commander gave him a clearance into the area. We were buffeted by the winds as Tim initiated a high orbit. "Air Ops IC, this is CALSTAR One," he squeezed in on the overburdened radio channel. "We are an EMS helicopter requested to fly into Grizzly Peak for evacuation of an injured firefighter. Please let us know when we are cleared into the area."

"CALSTAR One, we have you in sight. Be advised about three-minute delay before clearance into fire zone. We have a tanker run lined up. As soon as he's clear, we'll get you in."

Rose and I watched the aircraft swoop in and out of the smoke in seemingly random order. "Tim, how can we be sure we're not going to run into one of those guys?" I asked anxiously. "They want us right up on the peak."

Tim pointed to a small Cessna that was orbiting way above the smoke and confusion. "See that guy up there?" he asked. "He's the air boss—the guy I was just talking to. His whole job is to coordinate all the aircraft and make sure nobody runs into anyone. It's like having a moving air traffic control tower. But just the same, when we get cleared into the airspace, keep your heads up. There's a lot going on, and instructions can be misunderstood."

Eagle Five, the East Bay Regional Parks' helicopter, happened to be orbiting nearby. Tom, an ex-CALSTAR pilot, came
up on the radio to give us the lowdown on our LZ. "CALSTAR
One, this is Eagle One. Come up on Victor frequency." Tim
acknowledged, and switched over to a frequency that was
used pilot-to-pilot for unofficial business.

"Eagle Five, CALSTAR One. Is that you, Tom?"

"Hi, Tim, yeah. Listen, we were just into that LZ delivering
equipment and personnel. You will be landing on a ridge that
is just above Fish Ranch Road. There are wires to the south of
Highway 24, but otherwise no obstructions. The LZ is marked
by a fire truck, and the call sign is Engine 5357 on fire red."

"Eagle Five, just how close is the fire to the LZ? Got a couple of nurses here that are very interested in that information."

"Copy that, Tim. The fire is about half a mile away, and the
flank seemed to be under control when we were in. Unfortunately, the fire has jumped Highway 24 and is now spreading
toward Orinda. And with the winds it may be headed anywhere."

"Thanks for the info, Tom. Gotta go—the air boss just
cleared us into the area. Fly safe." We made a steep left bank
into the fire zone. "OK everybody," Tim said over the intercom, "heads up. Keep radio traffic to a minimum." There was
a strained silence as we headed to our LZ. We all knew exactly
where it was, as we drove along Highway 24 routinely. The
freeway had now been shut down, and flying up the empty
road I had taken to work earlier in the day was an eerie sight.

"Tim, I have our LZ on our right," Rosie said, pointing
through a blanket of smoke to a nearby ridge. A fire truck was
parked off to one side, and we could see the firefighter on the
ground giving us hand signals. The area did not appear to have
burned, and I couldn't see any flames nearby, much to our relief.

"Got it," Tim said. "Let dispatch know we're on short final."

As Tim settled the helicopter on the ground, the entire peak above us was engulfed in flames, spreading several miles in either direction. As soon as Tim cleared us out of the helicopter, Rose grabbed the scene bag and headed over to the firefighter who landed us, with me on her heels. She greeted him with a smile.

"Looks like you guys are pretty busy," she said. "Are they going to bring the patient here?"

The firefighter, who had his portable radio to his ear, motioned her to wait a minute. He listened intently, and then his hand dropped by his side. "The patient is dead," he said shortly. "They have to leave the body where it was found. But they're bringing you another guy that's hurt pretty bad. They'll be here in five minutes."

I stopped and looked around at the incredible scene surrounding us. The roar of the fire alone made conversation difficult; we had to shout to be heard. Occasionally another tree would burst into flames, providing a background of steady explosions. Above, and moving away from us, was a wall of flames, now sending smoke thousands of feet in the air. The hillside was already burnt out, and a crew of firefighters painstakingly moved over the steep terrain with hoses and shovels, suppressing any hot spots. A tanker flew by only a hundred feet above us, preparing to drop another load. For now the wind was blowing the smoke away from us, but it could change any time and trap us in this LZ.

The firefighter cocked his head, then pulled the radio up to his ear. "Hold on a sec, I'm getting an update on your patient." He listened intently for a few seconds, and I saw the expression on his face shift to one of deep anguish. "Never mind," he said, looking at the ground. "He's dead, too. They want to reposition you in the football field at Central High

School for staging. You'd better get out of here anyway. The way the wind is blowing, this fire could go anywhere."

Rose touched his arm. "I'm sorry," she said, and together we headed back to the helicopter. We were quickly cleared out of the area by the air boss, who then inquired about our fuel status. Since we had just completed the flight for the bicycle accident when we were activated for the fire, we hadn't had a chance to refuel. He directed us to Oakland Airport before stationing at Central High School. As we were cleared into Oakland, Tim gave us a rundown on how this was going to happen.

"You guys have never done a hot refuel, right? It's a little weird, but remember these guys do it all the time. We have to be quick to allow the next aircraft in—they need to stay in the air as much as possible before the sun goes down. Just stay buckled in your seat, and if there's any problem, be prepared to exit quickly. Like if there's a fire. But don't worry, these guys really know what they're doing."

"Tim," I said, "I know you're trying to make us feel better, but it's not helping."

"Just stay put and keep out of their way," he answered as we landed.

It was pretty scary. Two fire engines pulled up and trained their hoses on the helicopter. The fuel truck pulled up and within a minute they were pumping Jet A into the tanks—with our engines still running. As the refueler was finishing up and replacing the gas caps, Tim was pushing the throttle forward and we were in the air in seconds. I barely had time to glance out the door to make sure the gas cap was indeed on securely. The whole episode lasted less than five minutes.

"Pretty slick, huh?" Tim asked as we were airborne again heading toward the staging area.

"Actually," I replied. "I'd rather not do that again if we don't have to."

As we approached Central High from the Bay, the brisk winds blew all the smoke off to the west, giving us a clear picture of just how large the fire had become. The entire backdrop to Oakland was either on fire, or just smoking remnants of what used to be lovely homes. We all stared out the window, astonished by what we could see. Fire trucks and police cars at the edges of the fire looked like ants attacking an animal fifty times their size. Even to my uneducated eye, it was clear that things were wildly out of control.

We were asked to land in the football field and then come to the makeshift headquarters for a meeting at 4:00 p.m. to try and organize all our resources. When we were shut down, Tim stayed with the aircraft while Rose and I headed off to what was to be the first meeting of many that afternoon. The roar of the fire, along with regular explosions, still made talking difficult. The scene on the street was chaotic. Smoke filled the air and ashes fell steadily from the sky. Hundreds of people, many of them newly homeless, milled around, watching helplessly as their homes and businesses went up in flames.

The Red Cross was busy handing out coffee and sandwiches and setting up cots in the gymnasium for the displaced people. A semi truck from Safeway, a local grocery chain, pulled up and started an impromptu human chain to offload food and supplies for anyone who needed it. Down the street, the hamburger joint kept busy handing out burgers and fries to the disaster victims and workers. Firefighters from all over California were showing up on their own, carrying shovels, picks and axes, anxious to help.

After the meeting, we stood by at the helicopter, ready to go when needed. The plan was this: An ambulance would drive any serious casualty to the football field, and then we would fly them out to the closest appropriate facility. However, the news we got at that first meeting was that the smoke and fire were looming dangerously close to Children's Hospital, and they were considering evacuating all the patients—including the neonatal intensive care unit. Many of those tiny infants were too unstable to turn, much less be transported. Apparently, smoke was being sucked into the hospital's air vents, making it hazardous for both the patients and the staff. To make matters worse, I grimly reminded the incident commander, Children's did not have a helipad.

For the time being, there was nothing we could do but sit and wait. We collected some food and a Thermos of coffee, and camped out in the field, watching Oakland burn. Several times we were notified that we had a potential patient, but each time we were stood down. Either they were minor injuries, or they were dead. If they were dead, the police left the bodies where they lay to assist the coroner's office in the coming days. It was incredibly frustrating. Fortunately, though, the fire had taken a turn westward, and they didn't need to evacuate Children's after all.

The afternoon turned into night and as the sky darkened, the constant roar of the fire helicopters ceased, as they could no longer fly safely. A stillness settled onto our football field, punctuated by an occasional explosion, and the sky turned an eerie orange from the flames. The brisk wind finally died out, allowing the fire department to start getting the inferno contained.

At nine o'clock we were released. While the firefighters still had a long night ahead of them, the fear of major injuries had passed. We slowly gathered up our belongings and lifted off toward base. Everyone was very quiet. "What a day," Rosie remarked. "I think I want to go back to Tampa."

When we got back to quarters, it was time for a pilot change, and Pete was waiting to take over. Before he left, Tim hugged us both. "You guys realize there wasn't a damn thing you could have done for those firefighters. We did what we could." I knew that, but somehow it didn't seem like we'd done enough.

At 10:00 p.m., the phone rang. Rose answered it, expecting to be dispatched back to the fire. "Where in Oakland do they want us?"

"You're not going to Oakland," said Elise, our dispatcher. "You're headed to Half Moon Bay for a suspected SIDS."

We jogged out to the helicopter, belted in, and were off into the night sky. I was already emotionally drained from the disaster we had witnessed that day, and now we were going to pick up a victim of SIDS, or sudden infant death syndrome. I felt my brain go into automatic mode. I was going to have to concentrate on the mechanics of a full-blown code for an infant.

I hated these calls; they were usually horror shows. Most SIDS infants are long gone before anyone finds them, and we can do nothing for them. But they're babies, and we often carry on a code long after it's clear that the child is dead. After the baby is pronounced, our job is then to support the grieving parents. And that's the most difficult part of all.

As we headed for the coast, Rose reached over and squeezed my hand. "Are you OK to do this?" she asked. "If you want, I'll do primary."

"It doesn't matter. We'll both have a lot to do if this baby really is a full arrest. But I'm going to need you when this flight is over. Not a good day today." We were both quiet as we flew on, setting up our equipment and calculating drug doses.

We found the LZ easily as we passed the last ridgeline to the coast. After we landed, I grabbed the scene bag and headed for the ambulance, which pulled up as we landed. As soon as I opened the ambulance doors, I knew this was as bad as it could get. One paramedic was doing chest compressions with the infant on his lap. The baby wasn't intubated, and they had been unable to establish an IV—always difficult to do in infants. As I crawled in, they gave me a brief report.

"This is a two-month-old female that was found unresponsive by the grandparents about half an hour ago. She was a normal pregnancy and delivery, and apparently has been healthy until tonight. They started CPR right away, and fire was on scene in less than ten minutes. We've been unable to intubate her and can't find any IV access." While he was talking, I pulled out my equipment, preparing to intubate her while he talked. I gently inserted the laryngoscope blade into her mouth and was able to see the vocal cords. Unfortunately, a huge cascade of milk erupted from the esophagus, obscuring my view.

"Suction," I said urgently, holding out my hand while trying to keep a visual on the cords. Rose, who had just got into the ambulance, reached over, turned it on, and handed it to me. I gently suctioned out the baby's airway, and pushed the tube down through the cords into the trachea. I withdrew the blade and, still holding onto the tube, had the paramedic start bagging. We had good chest rise and could hear breath sounds.

As I taped the tube I said, "Rose, try and get an intra-osseous line. These guys haven't been able to find a vein, so let's not waste any more time. In the meantime, get me some epinephrine; we'll give it down the endotracheal tube. When you get the IO line established, we'll give a full round of drugs."

The paramedic handed me some drugs, which we squirted down the ETT. "We figure she's about five kilos," he said. He then hooked her up to their monitor. Not surprisingly, it showed asystole, or flat line.

"You guys ever have a heart rhythm?" I asked.

"No, nothing but asystole," he said. I looked out the back window of the ambulance and saw an elderly couple straining to see inside. They were clearly panic-stricken, and tears rolled down their cheeks. I nodded toward the window.

"Is that the family?" I asked the medic, who was reinforcing the tape on the endotracheal tube.

"It's the grandparents," he said. "They were babysitting while the mom and dad went out to dinner for the first time since she was born. They found her unresponsive in the crib and were absolutely frantic. They probably think they're responsible for all this. We tried to tell them this isn't their fault, but you know how that goes."

"We're going to Peninsula Hospital. Can you make sure they don't get into the car and try to drive over themselves?"

"Don't worry, we'll bring them."

"Great. Also, our flight time is only going to be about six minutes, so could you call ahead for report?" I asked, gathering up our stuff.

By this time, Rose had the intraosseous line established, and gave the first round of drugs. Predictably, there was no change. We laid our tiny patient on a backboard and prepared to load her into the helicopter. I looked over at Rose. She was focused on the child with an expression of deep anguish in her eyes. She glanced up at me. We both knew this child was dead.

Our flight over to Peninsula was quiet, with only murmured communication as we went through the motions of running the arrest. Not surprisingly, there was no response to our efforts. When we landed at the hospital, we unanimously decided to offload cold, or with the engines shut down. There was no point in endangering the staff under moving rotor blades. Rose brought a nurse over to do compressions while I carefully unhooked the baby from the monitors.

When we pulled into the ER, the team pulled out all the big guns, stopping only short of opening her chest for internal cardiac compressions. There was no response, and she was declared dead some twenty minutes later. In the meantime, the entire family had arrived, including the parents. They were quickly whisked away by pastoral care, but I still heard the screaming wail when the baby's mother heard the news. There is nothing quite as heart-wrenching as the cry of parents who discover their child has died.

One of the nurses came into the radio room where we were trying to chart. "We're going to be doing postmortem care in a minute. Would either of you like to come spend a few minutes with her before we send her to the morgue?" This was fairly common practice, particularly with children. We often only dealt with them in the middle of chaos, so it was a way to find some peace.

I looked at Rose. Her eyes were red and tearing, and she shook her head. "Can't do that," she said, and turned her head away. A tear slid down her cheek and blurred the ink on the chart.

I followed the nurse into the trauma room, and she left me alone with our tiny patient. She was lying on the gurney with the endotracheal tube and intraosseous line sticking out at unnatural angles. She was very pale and appeared to be sleeping. I gathered her up in my arms, taking care not to dislodge the lines. "I'm sorry," I said, gently stroking her head. "We tried everything we could, but we couldn't get you back. I'm so sorry." I rocked her for a while, crying silently as the events of the last twelve hours came flooding back. I gently laid her back on the bed and walked out of the room, shutting the door quietly behind me.

While we were flying home that night we could see the fire still smoldering in Oakland, but by now it was only red at the edges; there were no more hundred-foot sheets of flame. A huge patch of the Oakland Hills, normally covered with the small twinkling lights of homes, was now lit only by the glow of red emergency beacons.

CHAPTER THIRTEEN

Two Feet on the Ground

DURING the full ten years I flew with CALSTAR, I also spent time on the ground at Seton Medical Center in Daly City, where I worked in the emergency department. The day-to-day work wasn't quite as exciting as life in the helicopter—ninety-five percent of what we see in the ER is more or less clinic work. But that other five-percent can include some bizarre, pathetic and downright horrifying incidents.

One night I was working the evening shift, and I was feeling pretty low. The CALSTAR annual hangar party had been the previous night, with the theme "Life's a Beach." We all wore bad Hawaiian shirts or obnoxious surfin' dude outfits and swilled rum punch till the early hours of the morning. I had tried to call in sick, but a lack of staffing made that impossible. For the safety of the patients, I was relegated to the triage room, where my major responsibility was to take vital signs. Anyone remotely sick would be sent to the back immediately, and I wouldn't manage any critical care patients.

The shift had been a long one. I had triaged twenty shrill, screaming children, innumerable coughs and colds, and several obnoxious drunks, whose stench only reminded me of my own foolishness from the previous night. Overall, most of the patients were in better shape than I was.

At 11:30, I lay down on the couch in the "quiet room," which was usually reserved for counseling or grieving families. The waiting room had finally been cleared out, and I was impatiently watching the clock, praying for this hellish day to be over. Just when it seemed I might have made it, a car came careening into the ER parking lot and squealed to a stop—half on the sidewalk—right outside the window of the triage office. I ran out and found, to my horror, a white pickup truck with a man's head hanging out of the passenger window at an unnatural angle. Blood and brain tissue were smeared down the side of the truck.

The driver jumped out screaming, "You gotta help us! He's been shot! He's been shot!"

I turned to the security guard who had followed me out the door. "Quick," I told him, "go get a gurney and some help. Now. And tell them to bring an Ambubag."

"Got it," he said, and ran back into the department. I pulled on a pair of gloves and did a quick assessment of the patient. He had sustained several gunshot wounds to his head and had obvious gray matter oozing out of the jagged holes. He had only agonal respirations, very slow and irregular. He gazed forward out of unseeing eyes, and his pupils were fixed and dilated. He had a pulse, but it was very slow, probably in the thirties. I couldn't see any other bullet wounds to his torso or limbs, and I climbed into the driver's side and pulled him upright to initiate spinal precautions. I attempted to maneuver his jaw to open his airway, which was quickly filling with blood.

I found no radial or brachial pulses—meaning his blood pressure was less than sixty systolic. Reaching down to his groin, I tried to find a femoral pulse, but there was none. A woman sitting behind the seats was hysterical.

"They shot him! They shot him! Oh, my God, you have to help him," she screamed. By that time the entire ER staff had come running out, including the doc. We got the patient out of the car, placing him on a backboard, then onto the gurney. As we laid him flat, the blood that had been running out of his mouth began to pool in his airway, causing him to sputter and choke with each slow breath. We turned him on his side so the blood would trickle out rather than drown him. Then we ran into the trauma room, attempting to bag him manually.

He stopped breathing altogether as soon as we got into the room. The doc had him intubated right away, but it was too late. We knew this man wasn't going to live from the start, but we tried to get something back so at least he might be an organ donor.

According to the man and woman in the car, they had made a wrong turn as they left San Francisco and had ended up in a seedy part of town. A man had approached the car, demanding money. When they didn't comply, he took out a gun and shot the passenger several times at point blank range.

When the police arrived, however, another story emerged. These people hadn't mistakenly wandered into the wrong part of town; they had been told they could buy crack cocaine off the street in this area. The trio went into this dangerous area for the sole purpose of scoring drugs. They came across the wrong dealer, or maybe they couldn't agree on the terms of the deal. Either way, for this man it was the same outcome.

Like a neighborhood coffee shop, every ER has its regulars—or frequent fliers, as they are known—and Sylvia was one of ours. The ambulance radio report always went something like this:

"Seton, this is Medic 21 with Code 2 traffic. How do you copy?"

"This is Seton. Copy you 10-2. Go ahead with your traffic."

"Seton, we have a five-minute ETA to your facility with a seventy-year-old female with a chief complaint of altered level of consciousness. She was found lying on the floor of her apartment after a neighbor called in a welfare check to the police today. She had not been seen for three days. We found her with six empty vodka bottles, responsive to shaking only. She has extremely slurred speech, is unable to ambulate, and there is a strong odor of ETOH. She has been incontinent of both urine and feces, which is now dried to her skin. Her vital signs are stable. We are unable to elicit any past medical history from her due to her altered state, but she is well known to us. We believe you are quite familiar with her, too. Do you require any further?"

Nope. It could only be Sylvia.

All the nurses at the station tried to duck out the door, but Amber, the charge nurse, collared us. We suspiciously eyed one another, trying to come up with some excuse why we should not be the chosen one.

Regina was the first to speak up. "I got stuck with her last week. She hit me, bit me, and then slung shit at me. She was incontinent of stool five times. She pulled out her IV twice before we gave up. I've paid my dues for this month." With that she quickly ran into another room. I tried to be very small in the corner, just piece of furniture against the wall. It didn't work. My number was up.

Amber turned to me. "How long has it been for you?"

"Uh, about a month," I mumbled, realizing it was useless to protest.

The ambulance doors opened, and the breeze heralded the arrival of the great unwashed one. The paramedic, Karen, was wearing a mask and gloves and turning her head away from the smell. Sylvia's K-Mart nylon nightgown, soaked with unmentionable fluids, was dried to her skin.

"Hello, Sylvia," I managed. "How are you doing today?" Sylvia's only answer was a well-timed belch. We pulled her into the Rose Room, the ER's unofficial drunk tank. Out at the station, I could hear Edita, our unit clerk, setting up the obligatory pool so we could place bets on just how high Sylvia's blood alcohol was today. Edita had no formal medical training but somehow she always seemed to win these pools. I idly wondered how she got her inside line to the lab.

While struggling to get Sylvia undressed, I noted her slurred speech and the pervasive odor of stale vodka. Karen was cleaning up her gurney. "Hey, Karen, how many bottles did you find?"

"Six."

"Quarts or liters?"

"Liters, I think. Safeway house brand."

Quickly calculating this data, Sylvia's current condition, and my extensive knowledge of her drinking habits, I leaned my head out the door and yelled. "Edita, put me down for five bucks on 0.42." In California, legally drunk is 0.08; personally, I'd be staggering at 0.15.

Once we got the BA wagering set up and the money collected, my job was to clean up Sylvia. I hated this part. The human body produces any number of unpleasant byproducts, but my personal nemesis is feces. I can easily handle anything else—sputum, emesis, blood, urine, bile, the works. But the sight and smell of shit makes me gag. Frequently I would bribe other nurses if there were a bedpan involved with my patient.

Turning back to the task of making Sylvia presentable, I grabbed a mask and shook several drops of wintergreen oil near the nose. It wouldn't totally cover the stench, but it made it a bit more bearable. Decked out in battle gear of gown, double gloves and scented mask, I plunged into the first order of business: getting her undressed. It wasn't going to be easy. Her cheap nightgown, cemented to her skin by the dried feces and urine, stripped away her fragile skin as I tried to peel it off. Her perineum and buttocks were a mass of suppurating ulcers. She had really done it this time. She was a mess.

Sighing, I prepared the banana bag—an IV of folic acid, thiamine, magnesium and other choice ingredients that replace what the body has depleted from alcohol and poor diet. I hesitantly approached her with a basin of warm soapy water and prepared for the battle to come.

The way Sylvia saw it, she was sleeping peacefully when her nosy neighbor summoned the police. From her comfy alcoholic cocoon, she was grappled onto a gurney, dragged out into the frigid night, and dumped in the ER. Now there was this nurse sticking needles in her and trying to pull off her clothes. It was no wonder she did not take kindly to the bedbath. She made a credible attempt to punch me, but was unable to reach that far—her last drinking binge resulted in a broken shoulder from some unremembered fall, and it remained hugely swollen and purple. Thwarted, she tried to bite me but I was too quick. Besides, she'd lost her dentures months ago.

After forty-five minutes of struggling, I was able to breathe again. Sylvia glared at me, but was too spent to put up much of a fight. After setting her IV at 200 cc's per hour and restraining her hands, I placed a warming blanket over her and turned down the lights. Sylvia would be with us all night, taking up one room out of only twelve in the department. The most depressing part of all, I realized, is that this scene would be played out over and over again until one night, Sylvia would die, probably at home and alone.

Sylvia, when sober, was a delightful lady. Late one night, after hours of sobering her up, we sat down and had a long talk. She shared some of the happier moments of her life, and I came to realize she was a sweet, educated woman. For years she had worked as an accountant at a local firm, but was now retired and lived alone, barely surviving on social security and a minimal pension. Widowed and with no surviving family, her only companion was vodka, which was slowly destroying her body and mind. We had referred her to all the social services, including Alcoholics Anonymous and several self-help agencies, but she had thwarted all our efforts. The problem was that when she was sober she was quite capable of caring for herself, and she resented interference from the outside. She felt it was her own choice to drown herself in vodka, and it was nobody's business but her own.

Sylvia died at Seton Medical Center on May 16, 1994. The cause of death was a subdural hematoma, thought to be secondary to head trauma sustained in a fall while drinking, and complicated by multiple organ failure, exacerbated by chronic alcoholism.

No services were held.

I am always amazed by some people's inability to gauge the seriousness of a medical condition. On several occasions, we were summoned to the parking lot to "help get Grandma" out of the car. This was often followed by, "And she doesn't look so good." Occasionally, Grandma was a full arrest, and it's difficult to do chest compressions in the back seat of a two-door Honda. The family's reaction was often, "We thought she was sleeping." Oh, she's sleeping all right. And she's not going to wake up.

Then there are the macho men—the guys who are in disastrous denial. The story goes something like this: They start having chest pain, but ignore it. Initially, it's relatively mild, and rest usually relieves it. This goes on for several weeks or months. Then one day the pain won't go away, and it becomes so severe it is unbearable. Then the secondary stuff starts: They become pale and sweaty, then start vomiting. They realize they are having trouble breathing. About this time they can no longer hide it from their wives, who immediately insist on a trip to the emergency room. Of course, they want no part of doctors and hospitals, due to an intense suspicion that all things medical are some sort of scam. I think they see being sick as a sign of weakness.

So I'd be sitting in the triage room and a man would come stumbling in, clutching his chest, diaphoretic and retching— and clearly having a large heart attack. When I tried to get him into a wheelchair he would always protest, between labored breaths, "It's just a bad flu bug. You guys are overreacting. Really, just give me some antibiotics and I'll be fine." It isn't until he loses blood pressure and is in frank cardiogenic shock that he'll admit that this has been going on for a while, and yes, it does feel like a mule is sitting on his chest. The tragedy is if he had come in with the mild chest pain, he could have been treated easily, but now there's major, permanent damage. If he survives this event, only a percentage of his heart muscle will still be functioning, and he's become a cardiac cripple.

There is also a breed of patient in the ER who is incapable of understanding that someone else might need care more urgently than they do. Patience has never been one of my virtues, but sometimes it was all I could do to restrain myself.

One busy Saturday night, I found myself in charge of the ER. The wait to be seen was about two hours, and the mood in the waiting room was getting ugly. Patients who had managed to be placed in a room were now stalking the hallways, demanding attention. We were working as fast as we could, but the numbers were simply overwhelming our resources.

In the middle of this, we got an urgent call on the radio. "Seton, this is Medic 21 with Code 3 traffic, how do you copy?"

I reached for the radio. "This is Seton. Go ahead, Medic 21." I knew the caller well—Randy and his partner Dave had worked with us for many years. I trusted his judgment and his skills. He wasn't some hotshot Ricky Ranger who got a thrill running minor patients in Code 3. We could be assured this patient was critical.

"Seton, we have a four-minute ETA to your facility. On board we have an eighteen-year-old female, currently sixteen weeks pregnant with a chief complaint of severe abdominal pain and significant vaginal bleeding. She is a gravida five, para zero." That's four prior pregnancies, no live births. "She admits to alcohol and cocaine ingestion today," Randy continued, "and was involved with an altercation with her boyfriend, who assaulted her and kicked her repeatedly in the abdomen. She has heavy, bright red blood from her vagina, and we estimate blood loss in excess of two liters. How do you copy so far?"

I leaned over to Joan, one of my fellow nurses. "Get the OB/GYN room cleared out. And get one of the OB guys down here now. I don't care who. This lady is *sick*." Joan nodded and lifted the other phone. Over the radio transmission I could hear the patient yelling obscenities in the background. Her speech was slurred. "Medic 21, this is Seton. Copy you 10-2. Continue."

"Seton, continuing. Her last blood pressure is 70/38, and her heart rate is 160. She is pale, cool and diaphoretic. We have two large-bore IVs in place, wide open, and we believe delivery of the fetus is imminent. Do you require any further?"

"Medic 21, no. You're going into room five. Seton is clear."

I ran into the OB/GYN room to clear it for our patient's arrival. A sullen woman who was complaining about losing her place in line met me at the door. I tried to explain that we had a life-threatening emergency that needed to be in the room, but she was uninterested. "I've been waiting for two hours in this goddamn place," she fumed. "My sinuses are killing me. You people just don't care, do you?" She then hurled that cutting phrase we had all heard so many times before. "And you call yourselves an emergency room." She stamped out of the room, vowing to call the administration and let them know what a shoddy operation this was. Joan was at my elbow, watching this woman stalk away.

"What a selfish bitch," she muttered under her breath. "Anyway, Dr. Bates is on her way down, and I have the OR and lab coming over to help. I'll take her if you can help me get her started. OK?"

As usual, she had it all together. We watched as the doors opened and Randy and Dave pushed the gurney in at a run. Rivers of blood splashed onto the floor. Randy had not exaggerated in his report. We transferred her over to our gurney, and Dr. Bates headed south to try and stop the bright red blood gushing out between her legs. Her skin was a greenish gray, and she was barely conscious. Our ER doc got a central line started, while I placed another IV, got blood for labs, and prepared to run her over to the OR.

Dave helped as I hooked up the monitors. "She just delivered outside your door," he said. Randy had disappeared, I assumed, to start cleaning up the mess in the ambulance.

Dr. Bates looked up. "How many weeks was she?" she asked.

"Sixteen, according to dates. Not much chance for viability, huh?"

Dr. Bates shook her head and returned her attention to the bleeding. "Come on, we have to go to the OR for an emergency hysterectomy. Looks like a probable uterine rupture. She'll bleed to death if we don't get her over there pretty quick. Let's go."

Joan and the team pushed the gurney out the door toward the OR, leaving me in a room that only minutes earlier had been clean. Now blood was spattered over the floor and walls. I walked to the nursing station to call housekeeping, and I heard loud angry voices coming from the registrar's desk.

"Whaddya mean I can't go to the operating room to see her? I'd like to see you motherfuckers stop me." This was followed by a crash of furniture. I peered out the door to see security trying to wrestle a burly man to the floor. It was the boyfriend, obviously drunk and out of control. I didn't even try to get involved. I picked up the hotline to the Daly City Police to have them come and haul off this drunken oaf.

Returning to the OB/GYN room, I surveyed the mess. Randy hesitantly walked up to me carrying a small bloody bundle. He was shaking. "Uh, I don't know what to do with this," he said, depositing the bundle in my arm. "I just don't know what to do with this," he repeated and wiped a tear from his cheek. He turned abruptly and walked away.

I looked down at the bundle, knowing what it must be. I unwrapped it, expecting to see a cold, blue, and very dead baby. What I saw shocked me. Lying there was a tiny infant, about six inches long, still moving. It was so young that the skin was translucent, and the hands and feet were webbed. His eyes were still fused shut. I could clearly see all the internal organs, including lungs and a slowly beating heart. He was moving his arms and legs, attempting to gulp air. It was a little baby boy, otherwise perfectly formed with five little toes and fingers. I stood there, stunned. For the first time in my professional life, I had no idea what to do. This child had no chance of survival. And I couldn't stand the idea of the trauma involved in resuscitation.

Down the hall, the sinus woman caught sight of me. "Hey nurse," she screeched. "Hey bitch, I'm talking to you. When am I gonna get seen? Can't you people get anything right?"

Without responding to her, I turned and shut the door, laying the baby carefully down on the counter, which was covered with his mother's blood. I drew a basin of warm water and gently bathed him, taking care not to tear the paper-thin skin, then bundled him in warm blankets. I picked him up, and went and sat in the corner, gently rocking and singing to him while he struggled, clinging to life.

He finally died about ten minutes later. Joan had returned from the OR and hesitantly opened the door, surveying the scene. "He's gone," I said, and broke into tears. Together we rocked the baby.

"You take a few more minutes," she said as she got up and went to the door. "I'll take care of things out there."

I held the baby a while longer, then straightened my shoulders and headed back to deal with the woman with the sinus problems.

A Time to Die

Nurses are privileged to share in one of life's most significant moments—the moment of death. Some of these are peaceful, expected deaths; others are nightmares that leave us all shaken and speechless. There is a certain lovely rhythm in life; as the Bible says, a time to be born, and a time to die. Sharing these moments with patients and their families draws us into some of their most intimate experiences. This gives us, as nurses, a unique insight and perspective.

Most laypeople view death as inevitably tragic. I feel, quite to the contrary, that death is a natural part of life. It's the circumstances that can be tragic. I have spent time with elderly patients who know their death is approaching, and many look forward to being released from bodies that have been ravaged by time and disease. I was initially afraid of this aspect of nursing, and found myself being comforted by the very people I was supposedly caring for. From these people I've learned that death is often a peaceful process that can be likened to rebirth. Our task as nurses is not just to care for the dying, but to care for the family and help them cope with their loss.

I have also come to believe there is indeed life after death. As children, we are taken to church and taught that you go to this place called heaven after you die—if you were good. Most religions promise a life in the hereafter. There must be some reason everyone has come up with this story. And, after several encounters, I do believe it is true.

When I was working in the SICU, I cared for a relatively young man who had just had coronary artery bypass surgery. He had done well, right up to the time he had an unexpected cardiac arrest. Most of the staff were busy, so there were only four of us running the code. While we did so, I got the distinct impression that someone was sitting in the chair in the corner of the room. The feeling was so strong, I actually stopped doing compressions for a second to turn and look at who it was. There was no one there. The code was a quick one, and we got him back with relatively little intervention. As I was cleaning up, one of the other nurses pulled me into the corner.

"Did something weird happen here?" she asked. Initially I was reluctant to share what I had felt, but I couldn't deny it.

I didn't look at her directly. "Um, somebody was sitting in that chair over there." I looked up hesitantly, expecting her to laugh at me.

"So I didn't imagine it," she said. "I got the feeling he was watching us." She walked out of the room and we never discussed it again.

I had a similar experience several years later in the emergency room. An elderly Hispanic man was brought by ambulance in full arrest; he had been down for quite a while. The monitor showed asystole—no cardiac activity. As we were doing CPR, the patient took a deep breath and calmly folded his hands over his belly. We stopped CPR abruptly, checking to make sure the monitor was properly hooked up. The first rule of medicine is to treat the patient, not the monitors. All the leads were properly attached, and it still showed asystole. There were no pulses, so we continued the resuscitation.

About that time, I became aware of someone sitting on top of a six-foot cabinet in the corner of the room. I turned to look, but saw no one. Benny, the other nurse in the room, turned to look almost at the same time. We looked at each other, shrugged, and turned back to our work. We were unable to get this patient back, and after another fifteen minutes, the ER doc called it. Whoever or whatever had been sitting on the cabinet was gone.

As we were doing postmortem care and restocking the room, we were both uncharacteristically quiet. Benny broke the ice. "That guy was watching us, wasn't he?" she said, pointing to the cabinet.

"God, I thought it was just me," I said. "He was sitting on the top watching us, right?"

"That's the impression I got. I also got the feeling he didn't want to come back." And he hadn't.

Another patient in the SICU was actually able to relate his cardiac arrest to me. He too was a young man who had just come back from coronary bypass surgery. His graft began to leak, and he rapidly lost blood pressure. The surgeons came flying into the room, screaming for the wire cutters. After a sternotomy, the breastbone is literally wired back together, and they had to get the chest open quickly to evacuate the clot that had accumulated around his heart. The clot itself was compressing the heart, preventing it from filling. If it were not removed quickly, the heart muscle would have started to die from lack of oxygen.

The surgeon rapidly opened the chest incision, then snipped the wires holding the patient's sternum together. With a gloved hand, he reached into the chest and began open heart massage. To our collective horror, our patient's eyes began to flutter, then opened. He looked down to see the surgeon's hands in his open chest. The heart massage had been enough to circulate blood to his brain, and he was awake. We scrambled for some heavy sedation and wheeled him into the OR at a run, with the surgeon kneeling on the bed, continuing internal cardiac massage. They were able to fix the problem relatively easily, and he returned to the unit an hour later.

The next day when I got to work, our patient was sitting up in the chair trying to sip some apple juice through a straw. He regarded me thoughtfully. "You were the nurse that took care of me yesterday," he said thoughtfully. "Thanks. Guess I scared a few people."

I couldn't believe this man remembered me. He had not really woken up from his anesthesia when he coded. And he certainly hadn't woken up by the time I had gone home. How could he know my face?

"I only remember a little of yesterday," he said. "I remember having to make a choice to stay or go. It would have been much easier to just go, but I didn't want to leave my wife and kids." He spoke of feeling very peaceful; he wasn't afraid to go in the other direction. He simply felt he still had things to do and couldn't leave yet.

I do believe that people have something of a choice whether to leave or stay. We had a case on the helicopter where the patient clearly made the choice to live.

One summer afternoon Rose and I picked up a fourteen-year-old boy with a gunshot wound to his abdomen. He and his buddies had been playing with a loaded nine-millimeter and it had accidentally gone off into his belly at point-blank range. We landed at a schoolyard, where the ambulance was waiting for us. Rose was flying primary, and she headed off as soon as we landed. I followed soon after and found Rose packaging a very sick young man. His skin was greenish gray, and he was grossly diaphoretic—pale gray and sweaty, signs of someone in bad shock. He had only a thready femoral pulse, indicating a systolic blood pressure somewhere in the sixties. The paramedics had gotten two large-bore IVs in, and the patient was marginally awake. Rose looked up at me briefly. "We'll intubate him en route," she said. "He's got to get to the OR before he bleeds to death. Call John Muir and ask if we can go directly to the OR. And after I get him intubated, you get another IV, OK?" I nodded, and we prepared to load the patient into the helicopter.

After we were on our way, I helped Rose get out the intubation equipment and set up the monitors. As Rose inserted the tube nasally, I held cricoid pressure with one hand, and keyed up the radio with the other. "John Muir, CALSTAR One with Code 3 trauma traffic. How do you copy?"

"This is John Muir. Go ahead CALSTAR."

"We are currently en route with a nine-minute ETA. On board we have a fourteen-year-old male with an accidental gunshot wound to his umbilicus at point-blank range with a nine-millimeter handgun. His abdomen is grossly distended. His blood pressure is 68/32 with a heart rate of 143. His respiratory rate is thirty-six, and we are currently attempting a nasotracheal intubation. We would like to have the trauma team meet us at the helipad with blood, and take the patient directly to the OR, bypassing the ER. We realize this is an unusual request, but the patient is deteriorating rapidly."

There was a slight pause on the other end. "CALSTAR, John Muir. Will alert OR and have team standing by for you. John Muir is clear."

Rose slipped the tube into the trachea. Our patient was still awake, and she spoke to him quietly. "We had to put this tube in to help you breathe. I know it's uncomfortable, but we have to do this, OK?" He nodded slightly. He appeared to be fighting to stay awake. I turned my attention to getting another line started and wrapped a tourniquet tightly around his arm. "Hey, Rose," I said, not looking up. "Hand me a fourteen-gauge IV needle. He has a big vein over here." I held out my hand, expecting her to place the IV catheter in my hand. Rose didn't respond. I looked up, wondering what she might be doing. She was leaning over the patient and talking to him. I looked at the monitor. His blood pressure had dropped to 54/26.

By now, he was mostly unresponsive. I could hear her saying, "Come on, you have to hang in there. You gotta want to live. You have to hang on." His eyelids fluttered a bit, but there was no other response. I found myself becoming annoyed. This patient wasn't responsive because he had lost so much blood. We needed to pump fluids into him to get the blood pressure back up. And she was, I thought, wasting time talking.

I never did get that third IV started. The trauma team met us at the helipad as we requested, and we headed for the OR at a dead run. Our patient by that time had no blood pressure, and we had started chest compressions. Rose went up to the OR with them, and I returned to the helicopter to start cleaning up and to record the blood pressures from the monitor for our chart. I was startled to find one small, but significant increase in his BP—it corresponded exactly with the time of Rose's encouragement. I suddenly felt very small. I had gotten so wrapped up in the mechanical aspects of our care that I had forgotten the very essence of what we were trying to do.

Thankfully, the trauma team was able to locate and repair the damage quickly, and our patient did well. This young man owed his life to the entire EMS system, but I feel that a key to his survival was Rose's reassurance and encouragement. Because of her care, he made the decision in the helicopter that he was going to live. It would have been just as easy for him to let go.

Western medicine can't seem to accept death. A dying patient is often hidden in a guarded hospital room, and families are allowed in only periodically. When patients actually arrest, they are immediately ushered to a waiting room while the doctors and nurses run the code. If they're lucky, someone from pastoral care will sit with them until it's all over. The family is powerless to do anything but sit quietly and wait for the announcement from the doctor.

This is changing slowly, however. We are starting to allow families in while we're working on a patient, but there's a lot of resistance within the medical field. Though witnessing a code can be traumatic, it reassures families that we did everything possible, and it allows them to be present at the time of death. Some feel this helps them understand and cope with their loss. My own feelings are mixed—our interventions can be rather brutal and disfiguring, and if the code is a full-court press, it's a pretty busy place where we're moving fast. Adding a hysterical family member to the chaos could be distracting.

People often have unrealistic expectations of what medicine can or should do. "If you're sick, go to the doctor, and they'll fix you." Never mind that the patient is sixty pounds overweight, chain-smokes and has been slowly pickling himself with alcohol for years. Many people don't want to take responsibility for their bodies.

On the other hand, medicine *wants* to fix things. But the reality is we can't, and shouldn't, try to fix everybody. Human beings get sick and die. If we try to fix a person who is hopelessly ill, we are not doing any good. I always feel guilty and somewhat disgusted when performing compressions on a ninety-five-year-old, feeling their fragile ribs snap and crunch under my hands.

Families plead with us to *do something*. We want to act, to heal, to *do something* even in hopeless situations. But sometimes that means subjecting a dying patient to unnecessary, expensive torture. Some physicians—with varying intentions, and often fearful of litigation—will hold out to the family a glimmer of hope and offer heroic interventions. Frightened and unable to accept the inevitable, the family grabs on to this hope and ninety-year-old, senile Aunt Polly gets shipped off for a bypass operation. She never recovers and slowly dies in an ICU, in an alien place, in pain. And the family slips into a financial abyss trying to pay for it. Perhaps Aunt Polly would have been better served by remaining at home and dying peacefully with her family at her side.

The reality is, there are times when we shouldn't be trying to fix things. We need to recognize when it's time to allow nature to decide. At this point we become embroiled in an ethical and legal dilemma. And often we're forced to make these decisions when the situation is critical and there is little time for discussion or reflection. The public looks to the medical profession for guidance and, unfortunately, most of the time we choose to intervene. Once the process starts, it is almost impossible to stop it.

Marge was a typical example of well-intentioned medical care gone bad. She arrived at the emergency department one day with an acute heart attack and promptly arrested. Because she and her husband Ray had not discussed and planned for this, despite known extensive cardiovascular disease, we were obliged to resuscitate her. She came back, but was wildly unstable. She was admitted to the coronary care unit, and an intra-aortic balloon pump was inserted to augment her failing heart.

Ray was devastated by this turn of events. They had been married for forty years, and he felt he couldn't carry on without her. Her team of physicians carefully explained to him her poor prognosis in the face of cardiogenic shock and multi-system organ failure. Then one of them held out a last hope: If they did a bypass operation, she might get better. Ray did not hear the part of the discussion regarding risks, including the part that she probably would not survive the surgery, and if she did, she most certainly would suffer serious complications. He only heard that someone might save his beloved wife's life. Emotionally, he was not in any position to make a rational decision, and he insisted that everything be done for her.

To our dismay, Marge's name appeared on the OR schedule the next day. We half-heartedly set up an ICU room, not really expecting her to survive the surgery. To our surprise, she did return to us, but was as close to dead as anyone can be. She suffered a major stroke in the OR, as well as another heart attack. They were unable to wean her off the bypass machine, so she returned with her chest still open and still on partial bypass, as well as a balloon pump. She was on no fewer than fifteen drugs to augment her blood pressure. To add to this multi-system insult, her kidneys had shut down. We worked feverishly for her, and after two weeks finally got her stabilized.

But the operation had taken its toll. She was, for all intents, a potted plant from her stroke, never to be Marge again. She was on dialysis with no hope of ever regaining any kidney function. Dependent on the ventilator to breathe for her, her mouth and lips developed ulcers from the endotracheal tube, finally requiring a tracheostomy. Other tubes snaked in and out of every orifice to feed her and eliminate waste.

Ray was there every day for hours, talking to her, and helping us in her care. He was determined to never give up, even when confronted with the reality she would never be the same. In for a penny, in for a pound. One of the surgeons, too, refused to give up on her and continued to focus on the problem of the day, rather than trying to grasp the overall picture.

As time went on, Marge's pain increased. She lost circulation in her legs and we were forced to amputate them. First it was just toes, then feet, then below the knee, then above the knee up to the groin. She developed deep bedsores, as we had been unable to turn her for more than a week. So she returned to the OR again and again to debride the sores, and each time we gouged a little more out to rid her body of the necrotic tissue. Even though she had stroked, her nervous system was intact enough to feel pain. We gave her narcotics around the clock, and as time dragged on, she predictably developed a tolerance to the pain medication. It became harder and harder to keep her comfortable.

Finally, after three months of this nightmare, she coded and we were unable to get her back, much to our relief. Ray, now $900,000 in debt, was devastated by her death, but not bitter. He returned to the unit a week later with African violets for all the staff, to thank us for our work. We named ours Marge; it has thrived and grown into two huge plants. Every time I water them, I think of what we did to her and how disgusting it was.

This whole nightmarish scenario could have been avoided the day Marge hit the hospital. If someone had the integrity and the time to really sit down and discuss all the implications with Ray, all of this might have been averted. She could have died peacefully and quietly that day, rather than suffer terribly at our hands for the last three months of her life.

Marge's story should be enough to make people consider how they want to be managed if this occasion arises, and to write iron-clad instructions to dictate their wishes. Sometimes people do have honest and reasonable discussions with their families, but fail to follow this up with a written document. Most people don't realize that once the 911 system is activated, we are obliged to do everything possible until we receive a written no-code order from the patient's physician. Here's an example.

We received a seventy-four-year-old patient in the ER who was in the middle of a very large heart attack. His family was with him, and they were all uncharacteristically calm. "I know this is the big one," he said. "We've talked about this, and I don't want any heroic measures. All I want is for you to keep me comfortable." I felt very good about this and brought chairs into the room so they could be together.

"Do you have an advance directive?" I asked.

He shook his head. "Never got around to making one. But we're all pretty clear on this."

Glancing at his monitor, I realized this was going to be a problem. He was deteriorating, and without a written order from his doctor, we would be obliged to treat him as a full code. I discussed this with the ER doc, and we tried to contact this man's physician. Unfortunately, another doctor was taking calls for him and was unfamiliar with this patient. He was not comfortable writing a no-code order, having never met this man, and instructed me to contact the cardiologist on call that day. I agreed, hung up and paged Barry.

When he called back, I could tell Barry was having a bad day. I started to explain the situation, but he wasn't listening to me. We had interrupted his afternoon office hours and he was running way behind with a waiting room full of restless patients. "Admit him to the ICU," he barked. "I'll get there when I can." He slammed down the phone before I could get to the part about the patient's wishes. I figured we could keep things under control until he got there to write the no-code order, if it wasn't too long.

Fifteen minutes later, he came striding into the emergency room. "What's he still doing here?" he yelled at me. "I thought I told you to admit him to the ICU."

I tried to break into his tirade and explain. "He doesn't want—"

He cut me off. "I don't have time to discuss this with you now. Just get him to the unit."

"Look, Barry, he doesn't want any heroic efforts. And neither does his family. His blood pressure is only seventy now, and we don't have much time before we have to do something."

"Put him on a dopamine drip, and get him to the ICU. I'm not going to discuss this with you any further. I don't have the time. I've got to talk to the family," he said, and abruptly left the room.

If he wouldn't listen to me, I thought, he'd have to listen to the family. I started mixing up the dopamine drip, which would help increase his blood pressure, and asked the unit secretary to get me a bed. Unfortunately, there were no ICU beds available. I paged Barry overhead, determined to get all this hysteria toned down and make him listen to me. We needed to get this man and his family into a room upstairs, on the regular medical floor, so they could quietly come together in private.

When Barry got on the phone, it was obvious he had not listened to the family. He was yelling, "Why the hell is that patient still in the ER? I have to put in lines. What are you idiots *doing* down there?"

This put me over the edge. "Look, you're totally missing the point. This guy doesn't want—"

He cut me off again. "Just get him down here to the unit."

"Barry, even if I wanted to, we can't. There are no—." The phone went dead in my hands. "—ICU beds."

The family had gathered at our patient's bedside, and his condition was quickly deteriorating. I called the charge nurse in and explained the situation quietly in the corner. We decided to call the chief of cardiology, as he was a reasonable, level-headed man. Maybe he could rein in Barry. As I called the chief, ICU called to say they had transferred a patient to open up a bed.

Barry, now absolutely furious, showed up again in the ER. "Come on," he said. "I got them to open a bed in ICU." He grabbed a corner of the bed and started wheeling this poor man away. The patient and family were completely unaware that he intended to intubate this man and start placing invasive lines when he got to the ICU, both of which are unpleasant procedures. The family was following us down the hallway, and I didn't want them to see we were having a misunderstanding.

As we pulled this patient into the ICU, the family was out of earshot and I tried one last time. "Barry," I hissed. "You have to listen to me. This family doesn't want—"

"You've caused enough problems for one day," he interrupted. "You seem to be having a problem understanding I'm trying to save this man's life."

By now, the ICU staff had started moving the patient over

to his bed, and all I could do is back out the door. The machine was set in motion, and there was no stopping the chain of events. Despite the patient's wishes and family consensus, he was about to get exactly what he didn't want.

When the family found out what had happened, they were furious. Barry finally wrote that no-code order, the blood-pressure drugs were discontinued, and our patient died later that afternoon. Of course, this was after suffering at our hands for several hours. I have not yet forgiven Barry, or myself, for that day.

The Hardest Drive Home

O<small>H</small>, Lord, I didn't want to go. We had been out on a call until 3:00 a.m. Now it was five, and our dispatcher had awakened us after twenty minutes of sleep. We were to go to San Joaquin General to pick up a five-year-old girl who had been involved in a motor vehicle accident earlier in the evening. The mother, the dispatcher said, had been killed outright, and our patient had a head trauma, among other injuries, and needed to be transferred to Children's Oakland.

San Joaquin General is a small hospital near Stockton, serving mostly uninsured working-class patients in the Delta, a vast area of islands and irrigated farmland where the rivers that originate in the Sierra Nevada begin to converge on their way toward San Francisco Bay. When you fly over it you can see the extensive maze of levees that protect the low-lying areas from flooding and provide water for the farms. There are roads on top of these levees, and people often drive them too fast. There's also a lot of water-skiing in the Delta, as well as other activities that are often combined with drinking, so we were used to dealing with the resulting carnage.

Pushing the covers off, I staggered out of bed and struggled into my flight suit. It still smelled of blood and booze from our previous patient, a drunken highway crash victim who had puked on me. Outside, I could hear Tim already cranking up the helicopter. There was no way we would be getting back to sleep before the sun came up.

The ride to San Joaquin was quiet, each of us lost in our own reverie. Nobody was happy being up at this ungodly hour, and we knew this call was going to be difficult. It sounded as if this child was in serious trouble and needed to be at a pediatric trauma center yesterday.

According to our dispatcher's report, the girl was unconscious and posturing—that is, her body was intermittently stiffening, a sign that there is severe pressure building up in the brain. She had apparently begun having seizures that couldn't be controlled by the drugs they had tried in the hospital. She sounded like a very sick little girl.

As we landed at the hospital helipad, there was a barely perceptible lightening of the eastern sky, turning it from black to dark gray. The stars were beginning to fade, and the new day was on the horizon. Beth and I gathered our equipment, lashed it onto the litter, and looked in vain for someone to meet us with a gurney to help wheel our load into the hospital.

"This isn't good," I remarked. "Hope they just forgot about us and they're not too busy to come out."

Together we wrestled the litter out of the helicopter and trudged toward the hospital, an old and decrepit brick building. (It has since been updated.) When we got to emergency, we could see they hadn't forgotten about us—they were, as we feared, too busy. There was frantic activity everywhere. Telephones rang unanswered, staff dashed from room to room. I tried to grab a nurse as she ran by, but she shook me off, saying only, "In the major medical room."

"This is a fine hello," Beth said. "Want to guess which room she might be referring to?"

We put our litter down on the first unoccupied gurney we could find, an ancient, rusted thing with seized-up wheels that could only roll along at about half speed, and then started roaming from room to room, looking for a five-year-old trauma patient. When we peered around the corner of the main trauma room, a chaotic scene confronted us. There was a tiny infant, a little boy, lying on the bed, surrounded by white coats. The ER doctor, whose name tag said "Dr. Rubin," looked at us wearily. His face was gray from exhaustion, and blood was spattered over his wrinkled scrubs. I looked at the monitors—heart rate, blood pressure and blood oxygen—and they all told a bad story. When we edged our way into the room and next to the bed, we could see the baby's skin was mottled, a sign of shock, and his pupils were fixed and dilated. That means a severe head injury, or even brain death.

"I'm Janice from CALSTAR. This is Beth, my partner. Is this the patient we're transporting to Children's this morning?"

The information dispatch gave us was the best they could put together, but often they were relying on desperate second- and third-hand reports, and I could easily believe that a five-year-old female might turn out to be a three-month-old male.

"No, your kid is over in radiology getting a CT scan," the doctor replied. "This is the little brother of your patient. He just got here. He must have been thrown out of the car. Apparently, they found him an hour after the accident, lying in the reeds off the levee—the dad was so drunk he forgot to mention there was another child in the car, so nobody knew to look for him. The mother was pronounced dead at the scene. Can you guys take two critical patients with you to Children's, or should we activate another helicopter?"

"No, we can only take two patients if they are both relatively stable, and that certainly isn't the case here," said Beth.

Beth could make tough decisions fast and she was personable enough that people accepted them. We only had two caregivers on the helicopter, which sometimes was not enough for a critically ill patient; in a hospital emergency room the same patient might have five or more.

"Why don't you call Mediflight over in Modesto? They're only about twenty minutes away. But from the looks of this, I'm not real sure that child is going anywhere."

"Yeah, you may be right," he said, and turned to one of the nurses. "Get Children's on the phone and let them know we have another one that's probably brain-dead. Transfer the call in here so I can talk to the attending physician. And go ahead and activate Mediflight."

She nodded and left the room. He turned back to us. "Why don't you guys go over to your patient in CT and start assessing her. I don't have time right now to go over all of her history with you. I'll talk with you when she gets back here."

"OK," I said. "But where's the CT scanner?"

One of the nurses looked up from the IV she was trying to start. "I'm really sorry, we're all too busy to take you. But it's real easy to find. Just go to the main lobby, and it will be in the hallway off to your right. You can't miss it." Fair enough. After all, a CT scanner is a monstrous machine and it would be difficult to hide it. Beth and I looked at each other and headed out.

All the hospital's resources must have been concentrated on the little boy and his sister, and outside the trauma room it was dark and quiet. We pushed the squeaky old gurney through the tiled emergency area, which smelled of a thousand unwashed bodies. The early morning light was just entering the windows, adding to the surreal effect. When we reached the main lobby, a huge octagonal room, we found hallways branching out in eight different directions. There were no signs, and we stood in the pale light, like rats in a maze, trying to figure out which one of the hallways to our right might lead to the X-ray department, where the CT scanner would be.

"Might as well try this one," Beth suggested, her voice echoing, and we headed down one of the long quiet hallways.

The silence was suddenly broken by the hospital loud-speaker. "Code blue, CT scan. Code blue, CT scan." Code blue means cardiac arrest—someone was dying in the CT scanner. This announcement was a call for a pre-assigned team to respond immediately.

"Uh-oh." Beth looked at me in desperation. "You don't suppose this little hospital has two CT scans, do you?"

"That I doubt," I said as we picked up speed. Down at the end of the hall we had chosen, we found a very small sign reading "CT" and an arrow pointing down another hallway to our right. We could hear a commotion coming from a room at the end and figured we probably had stumbled into the right place.

The scene we found was about as bad as it can get. A little girl was on the CT table, with her head still in the scanner, and the attending nurse was attempting CPR. The only other person in the room was the tech, who was struggling to open the code cart, which contains the medication and emergency equipment to be used in a cardiac arrest. Technicians are trained to run the machines, not care for the patients, but there was no one else there—the only doctor and most of the nurses in the hospital were struggling to keep this patient's little brother alive over in the emergency department. As we came up to the table I looked at the EKG monitor, which showed a flat line, or asystole. This little girl's heart had stopped.

The hospital nurse and I pulled the girl away from the scanner so we could check her airway and get better access for chest compressions. Beth had already opened our med bag and quickly gave some epinephrine and atropine.

Meanwhile, I did a quick physical assessment. In addition to the breathing tube there was an IV in place. The little girl's arms and legs were intact, but her face was hugely swollen and bruised purple, and I could feel a large mushy area on the right side of her skull. Even in children, the skull is a pretty thick protective bone, and to find a large, unstable, depressed skull fracture is an indication of the force of the impact and indicates serious damage to the underlying brain tissue. By shining a light in the pupils, it's possible to get a ballpark estimate of the extent of brain damage—but her eyes were swollen shut from her injury, and I couldn't pry them open. A clear liquid streamed from her nose and ears, which I presumed was cerebral spinal fluid. That meant the sac enclosing the brain and spinal cord had been ruptured or penetrated in some way, probably by a bone fragment.

There were also abrasions across her chest and abdomen, and a section of the ribs was broken in more than one place—a flail segment. This injury carries a high risk of collapse of the underlying lung, and there was likely either air or blood escaping into the space containing the lungs and heart. Sure enough, the breath sounds were very faint and distant, indicating she probably had dropped that lung, leaving only one working. Her abdomen was tense, which indicated one or more of her major organs, perhaps the liver or spleen, had ruptured. The range of her injuries made her condition nearly hopeless.

The ER doc made it over to us and placed a chest tube. Although we got some improvement in the breath sounds, there was still no sign of cardiac activity after twenty minutes of aggressive treatment. We were still trying to get oxygen into her and keep her blood circulating with CPR. But the brain starts to die after three or four minutes without oxygen, and it had been at least twenty minutes after the accident before she was even picked up by the ambulance. She was probably brain-dead even before she reached the hospital. She might have survived the chest trauma alone, or the head trauma, or even the abdominal trauma, but when they were all added up, the result was inevitable.

As we worked, it became increasingly clear we weren't going to get anything back. We quietly discussed other options—such as opening up her chest and doing internal cardiac massage—but we all realized it would be futile, and I don't think any of us had the stomach to crack this poor child's chest open. We all knew what the score was.

We finally called it, the doctor quietly stating the time of death, and stepped back from the table. It was now light outside, and I could hear the morning birds singing. Our patient lay on the CT scanner table, still and pale, her face bloody and her body distorted from her injuries. The nursing supervisor would be notified to come and look after the body in preparation for the coroner's examination. We turned away and started to gather our equipment.

"So can you take the little brother, then?" the doc asked as we walked back toward the ER. "I mean you're here and all. Mediflight has a delay."

I looked at Beth. We were barely minutes from one pediatric arrest and death, and now we were faced with a critically ill baby. Emotionally battered and physically exhausted, I wasn't sure I had the strength to do it all over again. We glanced at each other, and sighed heavily. I gave her a hesitant nod.

"Of course," she said. "What's been happening to him while we were gone? He didn't look so good when we saw him last."

"No, he's not doing well. Got a bad head injury, too. He must also have either an occult bleed or a cardiac contusion, because he's pretty hypotensive, and on dopamine drip after a fifty-per-kilo bolus. I hated to give him so much fluid with his head injury, but you gotta prioritize. And he's also starting to ooze from everywhere, so I think he may be in early DIC—his platelet count is only 70,000. I've got a coagulation panel cooking now, and I've ordered FFP and platelets. He's also becoming harder to ventilate; his inspiratory pressures were getting into the fifties. When I left the ER, his heart rate was better, but not great."

Like his sister, this little boy had a disastrous combination of injuries. It was hard to imagine he could survive for any length of time, even if we could get him to Children's. However, as we pulled the grimy gurney along, I started my fluid and drug calculations. "How much does he weigh?" I asked.

"About nine kilos according to the Braslow tape," he answered. The Braslow tape is a laminated tape measure you lay alongside a child to make a quick estimate of his weight.

Overhead, the PA system boomed another message through the darkened hallways: "Dr. Rubin, return to the ER stat. Dr. Rubin, return to the ER stat."

"It's gotta be your kid," Dr. Rubin said, sprinting off. "Meet you over there. And hurry." We picked up our pace as much as the gurney would allow.

The PA blared again. "Code blue, emergency room. Code blue, emergency room."

"You don't think there might be another emergency room, do you?" Beth asked, panting as we ran down the dark corridors.

"No, I don't believe they would have two," I replied. We wheeled around the corner. Sure enough, in the trauma room, they were now doing compressions on the infant. The monitor showed asystole. We plunged in and did what we could to help.

"Do you want an ABG?" I asked. Arterial blood gas tests reveal the acidity and oxygenation level in the blood. Dr. Rubin nodded, and the nurse handed me the blood gas syringe. As I inserted the needle into the baby's groin, I gently drew blood—it was almost black, indicating little if any oxygenation, despite the fact he was being bagged with one-hundred-percent oxygen.

"This doesn't look good," I said. Arterial blood should be bright cherry red.

"Maybe it's venous," one of the nurses suggested.

"I don't think so," I answered. "It came up in the syringe with each compression. Who can take this and run it to the lab?"

"I'll take it over," said one of the paramedics who had brought the baby to the hospital and was still standing in the doorway.

Ten minutes later the lab telephoned with the ABGs. They were worse than horrible and indicated we had not gotten anywhere with our interventions.

Dr. Rubin sat back on a stool, defeated. "Anybody have any ideas?" he asked. No one answered. "OK, get Children's on the phone and see if they have any suggestions. If not, I think we're gonna have to call it."

I dialed up the ICU at Children's and got the attending physician on the line while the team continued their futile chest compressions. Dr. Rubin spoke quietly to the physician at Children's for a few minutes, then turned back to us, hanging up the phone.

"We'll call this at 6:59 a.m. Thank you all for your efforts." He turned and left the room. No one spoke. The nurse at the head of the bed cried quietly as she began to prepare the tiny body for the morgue.

Beth picked up the phone to call our dispatch. "James, it's Beth. Would you call the transport office at Children's and confirm that we won't be transporting either of these two patients? They're both dead. OK? Thanks. We'll be back in service as soon as we can get our supplies together."

She hung up and glanced at me. I felt a heaviness in my chest start to rise, threatening to spill into tears. I pushed them back down and quickly walked out to the ambulance bay to be alone. Beth walked out behind me with tears on her cheeks. We hugged each other quietly.

"We're zero for two this morning," she observed. "Not a real good start for the day."

We heard the full story later that week. The father had been out drinking and came home in a foul mood. He provoked a stormy argument with his wife, and for some unknown reason got the two kids up and put the whole family into the car. He was driving along a levee at over seventy miles per hour when he lost control. He was the only one to survive.

In our personal flights from hell, we all have a special dossier labeled "pediatric meningitis." Many of these children become desperately ill, despite early and aggressive medical intervention. There is an inexorable downward slide to septic shock—all the body systems speed up to the point where the various organs begin to fail. More often than not, it results in death.

We had been summoned by Children's Oakland to fly to Scenic General—a euphemistically named community hospital in the San Joaquin Valley—to pick up a three-year-old with a working diagnosis of meningiococcemia. As I asked questions and took the information from our dispatcher, my heart sank. Everything indicated a little kid who was rapidly deteriorating. Yes, his blood pressure was low, coupled with an astronomical heart rate. Yes, he was rapidly developing purpura, a purplish rash that quickly spreads and heralds the onset of disseminated intravascular coagulation (DIC) and profound, usually irreversible, septic shock. Yes, his respiratory rate was high, with poor arterial blood gases. And yes, all his blood work was markedly abnormal.

Deedee was my partner that day. Still fairly new to CAL-STAR, she had an extensive background in adult critical care and trauma but limited experience in pediatrics. She looked at me quizzically as I wrote down the clinical information.

"What are we going for?" she asked.

"Have you done a meningiococcemia yet?"

"What's that?"

"A particularly vicious form of meningitis."

"No, but it sounds like I'm about to."

Pete was our pilot. As we headed out into the valley, I pulled out my brain book, the small loose-leaf binder that we all carried in our flight suits. In it we kept up-to-date clinical information, drug dosages and other cheat sheets relating to the conditions we might encounter. Reverently, I opened it to the special section labeled "meningitis." I started with drug calculations, writing down a list of the correct doses.

With this type of meningitis, profound septic shock develops rapidly because children's bodies have not developed the compensatory mechanisms that adults have. A condition called third spacing occurs—fluids leak out of the blood vessels into the surrounding tissues and into the lungs. The metabolic processes increase and the patient begins to use enormous amounts of calories and oxygen. All the organs are affected and, as the demands overwhelm each function, they start failing with a fatal domino effect. Treatment for this condition is complex because we are trying to control contradictory conditions and because drug dosages often will be pushed dangerously high to support the blood pressure.

The closest we could land was a local airport, where an ambulance met us for a ten-minute drive. Scenic General looked like something out of a Hitchcock film. It's a county hospital that has always been run on a shoestring, but during the cutbacks of the eighties they had to pare down to the minimum. However, it's the only place in the county where the medical indigents receive acute care, and the hospital is always overflowing. Walking down the ER halls is like running the gauntlet, with people lying on rusting antique stretchers, reaching out to clutch at whoever passes by. The walls are painted that awful mint green so popular in the fifties, and it hasn't been touched since. There are no windows, just dank halls smelling of human excrement and years of disinfectant.

We were directed into the major medical room. The scene was as I had feared: There was a small child lying on a bed, deathly pale and covered with angry purple splotches. He was awake, terrified and intermittently crying for his mother who was on the other side of the room. His breathing was labored and it was clear he would soon lose consciousness. The team surrounding him was working feverishly, with trash littering the floor because they were too busy to get it into the garbage can. Nurses ran in and out, throwing the requested drugs and equipment onto the bed as everyone concentrated on the frightened little boy, while his mother hovered in the background, trying desperately to understand all the activity.

The doctor at the head of the bed looked up when we

walked into the room. I could have cried with relief. It was my old friend Val, who had been a physician in the pediatric ICU at Children's Oakland for years. I had heard rumors he had quit the high pressure of the ICU and moved out to the valley to help run a small pediatric clinic. We had worked together many times, and he was one of the best. He smiled as we walked in. "Janice, so glad to see you guys. Come on in."

The first priority in preparing the patient for the trip to Children's was to intubate him, despite the fact he was awake. Val and I discussed what we needed to do and got busy. Deedee started setting up our equipment, while mom was watching our every move. I left the bedside to introduce myself and tried to explain what we were about to do. I also wanted to get her out of the room while we performed some of the more invasive procedures—she didn't need to see the intubation—and she agreed to wait in the hallway. "May I just talk to him for a minute before he goes to sleep for the tube? I want him to know I'll be right outside."

"Of course," I said. "When we put the breathing tube in, we'll be giving him medicine to make him sleepy. But if you talk to him, he may hear you." She nodded and bravely walked up to the bed.

"Sweetheart, Mommy has to go and make a phone call to have Daddy come here to see you, OK? I'll be right outside." Gently she stroked his forehead.

"Mommy, wanna go home please," our little patient pleaded between labored breaths.

"Later, OK? I have to go call Daddy." I escorted her out to the hall, sobbing.

Two hours later, we had done all we could to try and stabilize this little boy. We had placed a central line and an arterial line to monitor blood pressure. We had given fluids, platelets and fresh frozen plasma, and had put him on three different drugs to help support his blood pressure. We had done all we could do to correct his wildly abnormal blood chemistries. We already had him on one-hundred-percent oxygen, but his blood oxygen level was heading south. And we had consulted the attending physician at Children's by phone many times, but the boy continued to deteriorate. We decided we could do no more at Scenic; we needed to get him to Children's. Once again, I thought, another child is dying before our eyes. And we can't stop it.

Val wished us luck as we climbed into the ambulance for the ride back to the airport. I figured it would be a minimum of forty-five minutes until we could push through the doors at Children's. The little boy was hanging in there for now, but forty-five minutes can be an eternity. We set out for the airport with lights and sirens.

As we reached the helicopter, we noted his heart rate climbing and his blood pressure dropping. I increased the dose of his vasopressors, the blood pressure drugs, and Deedee began pushing the fresh frozen plasma we had brought with us. Pete looked concerned. "He sure looks sick," he remarked as we quickly loaded our patient and ran the safety check.

"Pete, you have a real flair for noticing the obvious. Now get us the hell out of here."

We lifted off, and turning to our patient, I saw that increasing the vasopressors seemed to be helping the boy's condition a little. I relaxed slightly and started what would be at least a six-page chart. But soon the boy's heart rate started climbing again and his blood pressure slowly dipped. We pushed our drugs, but nothing was working. He finally lost his blood pressure altogether, and we started CPR. I got on the radio and called dispatch.

"Base, CALSTAR One. I need a stat phone patch to the pediatric ICU at Children's." I glanced at the cardiac monitor. His heart rate was now dropping to the thirties. Deedee pushed some atropine and epinephrine. Things were about to get really bad.

Luckily Andy was monitoring the CALSTAR dispatch radio. He quickly keyed up the mike. "Janice, this is Andy. I'm getting Children's on the phone now. Can I relay for you?" On a flight like this we regularly consulted the receiving hospital's attending physician, and the doctors at Children's were accustomed to seeing the patients through our eyes.

I quickly gave Andy an update to pass on to the doctor. "Tell her we're giving epinephrine, atropine and calcium. I've maxed the drips out. We've got no more room to go there. Tell her we'd like to start an epi-cal and an Isuprel drip as well. And find out if she's got any other ideas."

"Copy that, Janice. Stand by."

While Andy was calling the PICU, Deedee started mixing up the Isuprel and epi-cal while I continued compressions on the little boy's chest to keep his heart going.

"Pete," I called from the back, "can you make this thing go any faster?"

"Yeah, we're going into turbo mode," he answered, leaning forward in his seat. As if that was going to make us go any faster. "We have about twelve minutes to the Army base."

Andy called back a few minutes later. "I have the Children's physician on the phone. She concurs with your interventions. Start an epi-cal and Isuprel drip, and run them as fast as you need to get the heart rate and blood pressure up. Continue pushing fluids, colloids if possible."

"Copy that. Thanks, Andy." We got the new drugs started in addition to all the rest and, to our relief, his blood pressure and heart rate started to come up. We stopped compressions and began rapidly giving him more fluid.

One of the complicating factors in these transports was that Children's Oakland did not have a helipad at the time, so we had to land at Oakland Army Base and take another ten-minute ambulance ride to the hospital. As we were landing, the boy again lost his blood pressure. We reinitiated CPR and pushed the drips to even higher doses. Pete radioed our dispatch to apprise Children's that the patient had arrested again. We did a hot offload and moved him into the waiting ambulance.

During the ride to the hospital, we were able to get a cardiac rhythm back, but no pulses. We continued compressions all the way into the PICU. As we rolled the gurney through the door at a full run, the hospital staff was poised for action. We moved the boy off the stretcher over to the bed with CPR in progress.

It took almost half an hour to turn over care to the staff in the intensive care unit as we explained what we had done and identified the various IVs. As they took over, I sank gratefully into a chair, shaking.

Deedee slumped down beside me. "So this is meningio-coccemia."

We both knew this child didn't have much of a chance for survival. The drop in blood pressure and cardiac arrest had gone on for too long, and nothing was working, not even the big-gun drugs. Slowly we gathered our stuff and headed off to the helicopter.

When we got back to CALSTAR quarters, the new crew was waiting to take over and we discussed the case with them, trying to find a way we could have changed the outcome. We know we have to accept that sick people sometimes die, even with the most perfectly timed, flawless medical care. And sometimes those people happen to be kids. But this kid didn't deserve it. He never did anything to anyone. I wondered where God had been that morning, and why he had forgotten to care for this little boy.

As Deedee and I walked to our cars, she reached out and hugged me. "We did everything we could, you know," she said. "We all want him to live, but that doesn't always happen, you know?" She began to cry quietly, then abruptly turned away. "I gotta go home and hug my kids."

I got in my car and turned up the radio as loud as it would go, hoping to drown out the image of our patient lying on that bed, pleading for his mother to take him home. I started to shake uncontrollably and pulled over to the shoulder of the road where I started crying. How could something like this happen? Last night he was a normal healthy kid with a snotty nose, and now he was about to die. I realized I needed to be home with Mark. He'd help, he'd understand. I took a deep breath and pulled back into traffic.

After an eternity, I pushed the front door open. Mark was sitting in the living room, calmly reading the morning paper. I leaned against the door frame, defeated, and burst into tears. He came over and held me as I sobbed. "A little kid, right?" he asked. I nodded, and he held me, rocking me as I cried.

I didn't have to go back to CALSTAR for five days. The first thing I did when I returned was head for the follow-up folder to see how long this kid had hung in there before he died. I had prepared myself and now just wanted some closure. Harry came up behind me, anticipating my moves.

"Guess what?" he said. "Your kid is doing great. He was pretty sick for a few days, but now he's breathing on his own and giving them hell on the floor. He may even be going home next week. What do you think of that?"

What was there to say? Sometimes we can win.

Glossary

ABG: arterial blood gas

Alco: Alameda County

agonal respirations: a gasping, irregular breathing pattern that usually indicates death is imminent

Ambubag: a proprietary name for a manual breathing apparatus (*see* bagging)

arterial blood gas: a test to measure the levels of oxygen, carbon dioxide, pH and bicarbonate in a blood sample taken from an artery

aspiration pneumonia: a potentially fatal complication of pneumonia caused when food or fluid is inhaled into the lungs

asystole: no cardiac activity; indicated by a flat line on a cardiac monitor

BA: blood alcohol

backboard: a rigid body-length board with straps used to immobilize a patient during transport

bagging: manually assisting a patient's breathing using a polyvinyl bag connected to an oxygen source. A mask is attached and placed over the patient's mouth and nose to achieve a seal. The bag is then squeezed to force a breath in, and released to allow the patient to exhale.

BP: blood pressure

CDF: California Division of Forestry

cervical spine: the neck

CHP: California Highway Patrol

code: a cardiac arrest (in full, code blue); also refers to the sequence of procedures used to resuscitate a patient ("running the code"); also used as a verb ("the patient coded")

Code 2 traffic: a routine patient transfer

Code 3 traffic: transport of a seriously ill patient

CPR: cardiopulmonary resuscitation

cric: cricothyrotomy

cricoid pressure: pressure applied to the larynx on the front of the neck; it is applied during rapid sequence induction to prevent reflux or vomiting by the patient, which can cause aspiration pneumonia

cricothyrotomy: a procedure for establishing an emergency airway by making an incision in the cricothyroid membrane of the trachea and inserting an endotracheal tube

C-spine: cervical spine; the neck

diaphoretic: sweaty; one of the skin signs of shock

DIC: disseminated intravascular coagulation; a life-threatening condition caused by an abnormality in the blood's clotting factors

EKG: electrocardiogram

EMS: emergency medical services

endotracheal tube: a polyvinyl tube inserted via the mouth into the trachea to assist a patient's breathing

ETA: estimated time of arrival

ETCO$_2$: endotracheal carbon dioxide monitor; it detects CO$_2$ from each expiration and is used to ensure that an endotracheal tube has been properly placed in the trachea rather than the esophagus

ETOH: alcohol

ETT: endotracheal tube

FFP: fresh frozen plasma; a blood component that contains clotting factors

flail chest: an injury in which one or more ribs are fractured in two places, causing a floating rib segment, which compromises the integrity of the chest wall

GSW: gunshot wound

hypotensive: having a low blood pressure

IC: incident commander

ICU: intensive care unit

incident commander: a firefighter or police officer who is responsible for coordinating EMS activity at an accident scene

intubate: to insert a tube into the trachea in order to assist breathing

intraosseous line: a rigid needle inserted into bone to deliver emergency medications or fluids; used when unable to obtain an intravenous line in children up to six years of age.

IO: intraosseous

IV: intravenous

large-bore IV: an intravenous line with a large diameter, used to administer blood or fluid rapidly

laryngoscope: a lighted instrument used to aid the insertion of an endotrachael tube

LZ: landing zone

MCA: motorcycle accident

MI: myocardial infarction (heart attack)

MVA: motor vehicle accident

nasotracheal tube: a polyvinyl tube inserted via the nose into the trachea to assist a patient's breathing

OB/GYN: obstetrician/gynecologist

package: to prepare for transfer by placing the patient on a backboard, with a collar to immobilize the head and cervical spine; prevents aggravating any spinal injury and allows the patient to be moved in a controlled manner

perfusion: the flow of blood through the body

PICU: pediatric intensive care unit

RSI: rapid sequence induction

pleural decompression: the insertion of a needle into the chest wall to allow re-inflation of a collapsed lung.

posturing: a grave clinical finding that indicates pressure is building in the brain; the body goes rigid and the extremities are contorted

rapid sequence induction (RSI): a technique used to overcome airway reflexes (coughing, gagging, etc.) and prevent aspiration when intubating a conscious or semi-concious patient. It consists of preoxygenation, application of cricoid pressure and the administering of drugs that paralyze the muscles so there is no resistance to the laryngoscopy.

shock: a critical condition brought on by inadequate blood flow to the vital organs

septic shock: shock caused by infection

SICU: surgical intensive care unit

trauma bag: the backpack carried by a flight nurse to scene calls; it contains the equipment necessary for immediate care of the patient, including emergency airway supplies, cricothyrotomy kit, pleural decompression kit, IV supplies, bandaging and blood pressure cuffs

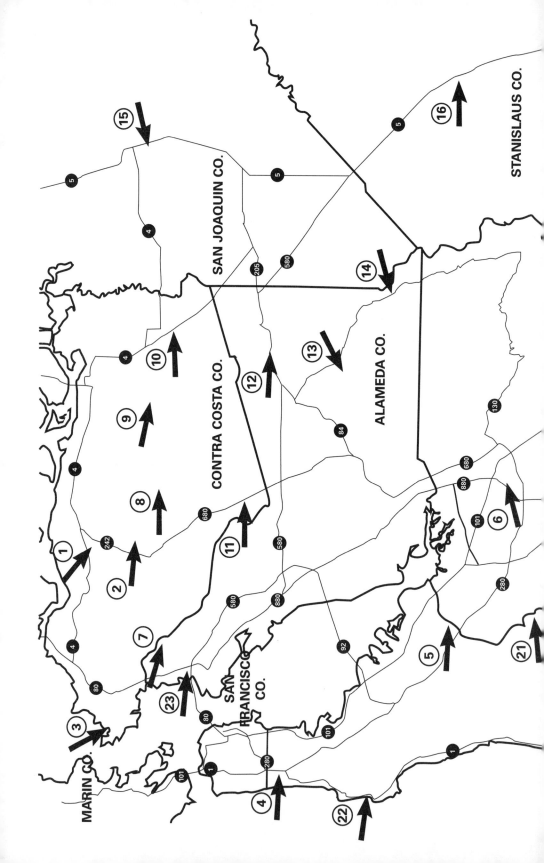

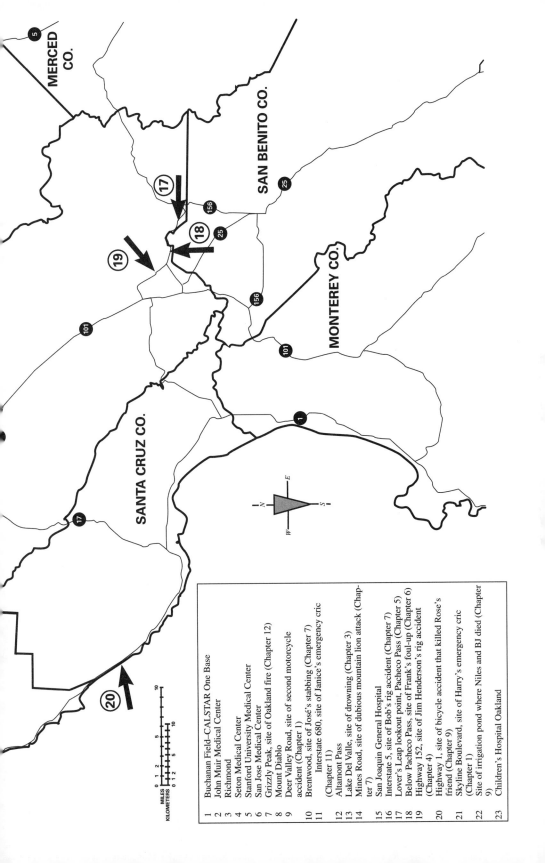

MILES
0 1 2   5   10
KILOMETERS
0 1 2 5   10

1   Buchanan Field–CALSTAR One Base
2   John Muir Medical Center
3   Richmond
4   Seton Medical Center
5   Stanford University Medical Center
6   San Jose Medical Center
7   Grizzly Peak, site of Oakland fire (Chapter 12)
8   Mount Diablo
9   Deer Valley Road, site of second motorcycle
      accident (Chapter 1)
10 Brentwood, site of José's stabbing (Chapter 7)
11 Interstate 680, site of Janice's emergency cric
      (Chapter 11)
12 Altamont Pass
13 Lake Del Valle, site of drowning (Chapter 3)
14 Mines Road, site of dubious mountain lion attack (Chap-
      ter 7)
15 San Joaquin General Hospital
16 Interstate 5, site of Bob's rig accident (Chapter 7)
17 Lover's Leap lookout point, Pacheco Pass (Chapter 5)
18 Below Pacheco Pass, site of Frank's foul-up (Chapter 6)
19 Highway 152, site of Jim Henderson's rig accident
      (Chapter 4)
20 Highway 1, site of bicycle accident that killed Rose's
      friend (Chapter 9)
21 Skyline Boulevard, site of Harry's emergency cric
      (Chapter 1)
22 Site of irrigation pond where Niles and BJ died (Chapter
      9)
23 Children's Hospital Oakland